T0266300

# Sensitive

# Sensitive

my journey through

a toxic world

## Pookie Sekmet

She Writes Press

Copyright © 2019 by Pookie Sekmet

All rights reserved. No part of this publication may be reproduced, distributed, or transmitted in any form or by any means, including photocopying, recording, digital scanning, or other electronic or mechanical methods, without the prior written permission of the publisher, except in the case of brief quotations embodied in critical reviews and certain other noncommercial uses permitted by copyright law. For permission requests, please address She Writes Press.

Published October 2019
Printed in the United States of America
Print ISBN: 978-1-63152-618-3
E-ISBN: 978-1-63152-619-0
Library of Congress Control Number: 2019912234

Interior design by Tabitha Lahr

For information, address:
She Writes Press
1569 Solano Ave #546
Berkeley, CA 94707

She Writes Press is a division of SparkPoint Studio, LLC.

Names and identifying characteristics have been changed to protect the privacy of certain individuals.

# Contents

∽

# Introduction

∾

Gentle reader, I can help you. I have knowledge not otherwise available about the contaminants and toxins in your everyday life. I see our world clearly, and I will tell you what I see. At the same time, I will tell a parallel story about my own life so that when you learn the price I paid for clarity and wisdom, you will trust that my voice is a true one.

Seven years ago I was incapacitated by intolerance to fragrances and other common chemicals, and even now I am impaired. Due to my illness, I have lost vocabulary. But the disabled also have important stories to tell, and I have found the words to tell this story.

I am a middle-aged white woman and my malady has made me unemployable. I groom myself without flair and wear undistinguished clothing. Sometimes I walk the single long block from my house to the post office wearing the same pilled charcoal gray hoodie and dark plaid pajama bottoms that I just slept in. Such is the tolerant nature of my small Western Massachusetts town that I do not feel judged for my appearance. I have lived in this town for only a few years, but I am happy here in a way I haven't been since childhood.

I am lucky in this local acceptance of oddity because I carry with me, wherever I go, a half facepiece cartridge respirator that looks sort of like a gas mask. The cartridges keep out many common airborne chemicals and fragrances, so I put it on before entering the post office or library, or if a diesel truck drives by, or if someone who has used dryer sheets passes near me. People in this kindhearted town might do an inadvertent double take, but their expressions remain friendly and they do not stare. If people cannot see your face, at a subconscious level they worry there is something wrong with you. Sometimes I am sad there is a barrier between me and these lovely people, but the reality is that I am broken and their subconscious suspicions are correct.

One day in 1964 when I was a baby, my parents found me unresponsive. They rushed me to the hospital, and the doctors thought I was dying. I was in a coma for several days, and I stayed in the hospital for several weeks. After my parents took me home, it was close to a year before I explored my environment as I had before the illness, and, for many years afterward, I was an unusually quiet and reserved child. The few times this event was discussed within the family, my parents told me that the doctors were never sure what had caused the illness.

My whole life I had fatigue, bad sleep, noise sensitivity, and lack of physical stamina. Sometimes there were periods of nonspecific ill health that were more acute. Despite academic accomplishment, I left college twice abruptly, and, despite professional promise, I left jobs abruptly many times. I was fired from jobs for episodes of disconcerting behavior. I had trouble maintaining friendships. For long periods my life was a painful and exhausting struggle. Neither I nor anyone around me ever made a connection between my impairments and the early illness.

Then, in 2010, when I was forty-eight and working as a mid-level accountant, I became seriously ill from a job workspace I had just moved into. Over the next few years, as I struggled to carry on while suffering terrible neurological symptoms including extreme fatigue and insomnia, loss of memory, inability to find words, depression, and the inability to recognize common objects, I finally pieced the puzzle together. The illness when I was a baby must have been from a chemical exposure, which weakened my nervous system and other aspects of my health and created an underlying chemical intolerance. The toxic job in 2010 forced me to solve this mystery, but the repeated exposures in that workspace gave my nervous system a second, severe, and, this time, crippling chemical injury. I was left with a new and permanent intolerance to chemicals commonly found in just about every car, workplace, shop, mall, theater, restaurant, medical facility, government office, and mode of transport. Now I am largely housebound, and even at home I must be careful about exposures to incoming mail, cleaning products, dust, personal care products, and food additives.

I see the world more clearly than other people, and I mean the actual, tangible world. Other people contentedly get into their cars, but I see toxic boxes on wheels conveying hapless families who are unwittingly ingesting damaging gasses from interior car components. I stop to chat with a neighbor who smells of laundry products, and I see a hormone-disrupting cloud emanating from her clothing and attached to her wherever she goes. Looking at a photo of new housing, I see commercial-grade paint, caulk, and plywood all oozing volatile organic compounds, carpets oozing formaldehyde and off-gassing glues, and sofas and soft furnishings oozing formaldehyde and other toxic chemicals. In advertisements for air fresheners or laundry scents, I see pure cynical evil. There is no one minding the shop, meaning to a great extent no one is ensuring that our products are safe.

I want to tell my story and help others see their environments at work, home, and school more clearly. I want to make some sense of my life so far. I know I must stay home so that I'm not made ill, and I must find contentment and joy within the constraints of my disability. Part of my contentment will come from sharing what I have paid such a high price to learn: that there are invisible toxins all around us that are changing us as organisms and as people.

# Chapter 1 - The Questions

After decades of illness, sometimes low-level and sometimes acute, I finally have more days of wellness than days of illness. This current period of relative health has freed my mind from the linked imperatives of managing my illness and struggling to survive. Now I can consider what I want to do during the rest of my life and who I can yet become. When I am ill, in addition to feeling awful, I am burdened by the sense that this life is passing while I am a sad shadow of my true self. And I have been ill so much that I don't know who I am anymore. What are the core qualities that I still possess, that are truly of me, that can define a future life of happiness and joy?

If my problem had only been family emotional trauma, of which there was plenty, I believe my native gifts of resilience, cheerfulness, and creativity would have allowed me to have a full life. Had I not received the neurological injury as an infant and had I instead possessed basic health, I would have traveled widely and made many friends. I would have been extremely fit. I would have had a rich career with the usual bumps due to gender-based societal bias, and I would have had children.

Instead, in addition to having troubled relationships with family members, I repeatedly became impaired from exposures to different home and work environments. The impairments manifested as a collection of chronic symptoms that were never properly diagnosed but were instead attributed by my parents to character weakness and vague personality deficiencies. Many people have immediate and temporary adverse environmental responses, such as from allergies. With me, the effects of an environmental exposure were delayed, long-lasting, and, until 2010, subtle. Since my early teens, I also had severe premenstrual symptoms and debilitating menstrual pain, which my parents blamed on my inability to manage my own stress and anxiety. I now know that the painful menstruation was also caused by the neurological and adrenal damage I suffered as a baby. Because my nervous system needed a long time to recover from any particular exposure, because the exposures were overlapping and the effects were delayed, and because there was an additional layer of pain and fatigue caused by my monthly period, it was impossible for me to connect the dots and identify what was wrong.

The exposures compromised my nervous system, including brain function. During the occasional episodes prior to 2010 when I was more acutely ill, I lost memory, language, and the cognitive ability to accurately self-assess and self-diagnose. Doctors never grasped the whole picture. As years passed, despite making good grades in school and then working hard in jobs, I was unable to achieve contentment and ease because I slept badly and felt ill to some degree almost all of the time. Long-term fatigue and malaise gave me chronic low-level anxiety and probably low-level depression. Despite my affection for my family and my calm determination to achieve scholastic and professional success, my parents followed a script in which any misfortunes I suffered were due to my own emotional and psychological weaknesses. Because I was ill so much, my connection to the world was tenuous, as if there wasn't a place for me in it.

Instead of seeing myself as psychologically impaired, I need to see myself with extreme and disciplined clarity as someone whose true nature and capacity for wholeness are destroyed by environmental toxins. These exposures are the enemy of my true self. When I have an adverse exposure, my core is eroded just as water erodes a riverbank. We are all temporary lumps of flesh in a chemical soup, but for me there is no shell to protect me from the chemicals, which enter my body and immediately disrupt my neurological balance and make me ill, tired, and brain foggy. This injury defines me. My existence will be garbage and my entire life will be a wasteland of despair if I continue to be ill as I have been in the past. I can never have a normal life and must instead dig deep for what self-determination and strength I have left, to build an unconventional new life according to my own rules.

My condition is not widely understood, and only recently have doctors been persuaded by my self-diagnosis. The term multiple chemical sensitivities (MCS) is often used for debilitating conditions that have their roots in allergic reaction, but my own condition has never been associated with an allergic response and is instead a result of a single severe chemical exposure. This initial triggering chemical exposure damaged my nervous system and, in combination with later exposures, ultimately gave me a broad-based intolerance to fairly low levels of fragrance and other common chemicals. Under the umbrella of MCS, the best specific description for my condition is probably *toxicant-induced loss of tolerance*—TILT, a term coined by Dr. Claudia Miller. In this book, I have shortened this term to simply "chemical intolerance."

Can I look back to a time when I was whole? My early high school years were the last time I felt truly alive and free of the sense that life was at least some degree of burdensome struggle. Back then I was accepting, accommodating of the foibles of others, and unquestioning of my parents' hands-off approach to raising their children. Because my intentions were good, I believed in the good intentions of people around me. I felt safe, not necessarily every day in our home, but in the future because I believed that the love within the family and the basic goodness of its members would persevere intact. I saw a future with these people. It seems contradictory that at a time of family turmoil I could have been happy and content, but I thought the upheavals were only temporary hiccups within our superior clan.

There were aspects of my parents' lives, like their clothes, hobbies, financial status, or how they talked to each other or to my siblings, that I noticed but believed were none of my business. Whereas then I did not judge or interpret these details, now I know they are truth signifiers. If I want to understand who I can yet be after the devastation of my illness, I need to understand who I was before I became ill. I need to study the snapshots, read the letters and other documentation, and remember signs and signals that I previously ignored. Then I can answer questions that never occurred to me until I became so ill when I was forty-eight. Did my family keep information from me that could have helped me manage my illness, decades before it crippled me? Their disregard is obvious to me now, but it wasn't then. What were the reasons for this disregard? I have lost so much throughout my life. Were these the people who took it from me?

People close to either the beginning or the end of their lives seem less attached to life and also less attached to people around them. We are more inclined to accept vague explanations for the mechanics of their passing over. No one knew exactly why my father died in his early eighties, and, if my seventy-four-year-old husband died tomorrow, despite his glossy and robust bulk I doubt anyone would feel compelled to cut him open and root around inside looking for an explanation. Babies often die from mysterious or falsely attributed causes. What is the point of teasing apart that tender and sad dead flesh to put a technical label on such a tragedy? Better to gloss it over with a vague explanation, and let the bereaved parents go home to lick their wounds and tend to their living offspring.

In mid-1964, when a clean-cut, well-spoken couple took their limp baby to a university-affiliated hospital in Toronto and told the doctors that they had no idea what had happened, no one disbelieved them. My mother and father were appropriately distraught, and I showed no signs of physical abuse. This sad event would just be yet another mysterious infant death with no lessons to be learned, the doctors thought.

At the time of my illness, my father had a fledgling academic career as a history professor and my pregnant mother was working toward a doctorate degree in psychology. Although they had both suffered traumas and losses during childhood, they had built a strong marriage, had many friends, were both extremely healthy, and looked forward to vibrant professional lives. I now believe it is possible that between the time Mom and Dad found that I was ill and the time they delivered me to the medical professionals, my parents concocted a cover story for what they thought would be my death. According to this theory, when they found me, they also recognized with horror within our living space the chemical that had poisoned me. Why incur permanent social shame and career damage from admitting that your negligence killed your child, if the child is already a write-off because it is almost a certainty she will die?

My second theory is that initially they didn't know the cause; therefore, they didn't lie to the doctors in those first moments. This second theory has them figuring out the true cause at a later date. The first theory depends on them being almost certain I would die, because if there were a chance that revealing the true cause could have helped the doctors save me, my parents would have confessed. If, on the other hand, they only suspected the cause at first and became convinced of it later, after I emerged from the coma for example, or even after a few years during which I seemed fine, then at that point there would have been no point to admitting the truth. I was better, wasn't I? I will never know and will not try to prove which of these scenarios is true. The lie is the important feature, whether it occurred immediately or at a later time.

Now that I have diagnosed my illness and learned to manage it by staying home to avoid the chemicals that make me ill, my new relative health and mental strength have given me a fresh view. If I can prove that my parents hid the true cause of my childhood illness, then I can repudiate their explanations for my disrupted past life. If I can prove to myself that they lied, then I will know it wasn't my mind that was impaired for all those years—it was my body. I didn't leave college repeatedly, lose jobs, and have friendships fall away because my personality was damaged or weak. These things happened because I was ill. If I can recast my past, I will claim a place for myself in the world.

I don't have much concrete evidence of their lie, just a few fragments from long-ago conversations. I must instead dig deep into old relationships and impressions. It is painful, even vaguely nasty feeling, to go back and pick off old scabs, shift around old wormy shite. But I have never been afraid of heavy lifting or a dirty job. I can bounce back from this.

# Chapter 2 - The Big Life

In his prime, which lasted many decades, my father had the look of a shorter, more leanly muscular, and more handsome Cary Grant. He had a movie star's ability to gather the attention of others to himself, and he never doubted that this attention was justified. I inherited from Dad the tendency to have several ambitious projects cooking at the same time, the ability to think strategically and on a large scale, and an absolute absence of laziness. Like him, I don't think the usual rules apply to me, although the two of us expressed this personal belief in vastly different life choices.

Dad liked to show off his beauty and physical prowess. There are many snapshots of him holding one of his babies high above his head with one hand, both baby and father laughing with delight. He loved to throw naked babies in the air and catch them. My father liked to be around other attractive people. Early in his marriage, when he and Mom got together with couples who were friends of theirs, they would all meet at parks, beaches, and playing fields so the men could play frisbee. The men were trim and tan with short hair, and they took off their shirts in the sun. Think Southern California young academics in the early 1960s, meaning chinos, low-profile sneakers, and white T-shirts or white collared shirts for the men, and effortless, pretty, gathered dresses for the women. While the men hurled the frisbees across great distances with a lot of yelling, encouraging each other's showmanship, their women sat on blankets, looking like flowers and tending to the food and the babies. No hippy style yet; not ever for my dad, who for his whole life maintained a classic look.

Bicycles were a passion for many athletic young men of that time and place, and my father developed a lifelong love of distance bike riding. Since he had the flexibility of an academic schedule and Mom to look after things at home, one summer he was able to take time off and ride a bicycle by himself across the country from California to coastal North Carolina. Then later, he rode down the West Coast from Canada to Mexico, and a few years after that up the East Coast from Key West to the tip of Maine; in his early middle age, he rode across the country from East to West. When the family all lived together, he frequently came home with scrapes and bruises from falling off his bicycle. I have no memory of him wearing a helmet during those years.

By the time my parents had four children under the age of eight, they had settled in a university town in the Deep South, where Dad had a tenure-track job teaching history and Mom was a psychologist. Dad continued his exuberant lifestyle. He loved "the car auction," a local institution, and came home with curiosities like a WWII-era military troop bus shaped like a large beetle, a Korean War–era ambulance, and a stylish red bench-seat convertible. In the early years, he also loved motorcycles. For everyday use, he bought cars of dubious mechanical reliability at the auction for almost no money and then "fixed" them himself. Throughout my childhood we pushed these clunkers down the street when they wouldn't start, Dad running along and pushing from the driver's doorway while steering with one hand and then jumping in when the engine turned over, all with loud shouts and flourishes. Mom's mother came for a visit when Mom was pregnant with my younger sister, Amy, and Dad was delighted later when my older sister, Kirsten, told the story of Grandma's horror when Mom helped to push a car down the street, leaning forward with her large belly hanging. For Dad, the retelling of this story celebrated our virtuous eccentricity as a family. Another time when he was by himself in a car, the brakes failed while he was going downhill. He lost some teeth when he had to stop the car by driving it into some bushes. This story was not celebrated. I don't remember ever using seatbelts as a child.

Dad dressed beautifully, in a sort of Brooks Brothers meets luxury bohemian style, and whether he was at leisure in jeans and a T-shirt, giving a lecture in jacket and tie, or on a long run with a buddy, he always looked like five million bucks. He bought himself camera equipment, nice watches, stereo components, classical music records, and art books. Since there weren't enough calories or high-protein groceries in our house to support his exercise regimen, he ate large lunches by himself or sometimes with a colleague in pleasant local venues like the university faculty club, a steakhouse, or a seafood restaurant.

Dad had a keen eye for quality in decorative objects, rugs, and furniture. Our homes weren't large, but the common rooms were elegant in the Arts and Crafts style, with oak floors, large, richly colored oriental rugs, dark furniture, and golden glowing area lights.

My father had an aggressively adventurous spirit and believed he could live large in the world, not through overconsumption, but in terms of working hard, planning hard, and grabbing large opportunities as they presented themselves. He was able to discern and exploit hidden value in assets that he acquired for little money. When I was about ten years old, he began to buy investment properties in our hometown, starting with a four-unit apartment building across the street from our house. Even though he and Mom didn't make large salaries, he was good at saving money and had opportunities over time to purchase individual houses or small multiunit buildings to advantage. He intuited the power of positive cash flow and leverage in the very early 1970s, long before the explosion of published real estate wealth-building guidance.

Around 1975, he learned that the university wanted to off-load a beautiful and well-built seven-unit apartment building that was right on campus. He worked out a deal where his collection of early twentieth-century art glass and pottery, acquired for low prices in junk stores, would go to the university's art museum as one-sixth of the purchase price, in partial exchange for the building—Tiffany, Rookwood, Grueby, all that shit. This elegant piece of real estate, acquired for no cash down, threw off wheelbarrows of cash for many years, funding his children's higher educations and his own longer-term wealth.

He wrote and published many books, competed in many marathons and triathlons, and spoke several European languages. He traveled solo widely, often swinging through Brooks Brothers in New York City when he was en route to or from Europe. In addition to the art glass and pottery, he accumulated other strategic investments in the form of art collections: bronzes from around the turn of the twentieth century that he bought in European auction houses and antique and vintage ethnic textiles. In late middle age, he started prospecting for a certain type of jade that he found in riverbeds in Central America. He traveled to a remote jungle region dozens of times, and to find this jade he made long treks into the bush accompanied by hired men with large and visible guns, and burros to carry out the rocks.

My father wanted to see himself as in command of his life, able to go anywhere and do anything. In his self-focus, he did not reach out to his children to teach them or help them to have large lives like his. His pursuits were solitary. Whatever he learned from his adventures, he kept to himself.

After Dad's death, my brother, Hunter, and I conjectured that his late-life dementia had been caused by the repeated blunt-force traumas to his head from bicycle accidents, car accidents, and other random impacts from his active life. He was often gesturally impulsive when executing a repair around the house or to his vehicles and was not careful with chemicals or dusts. He had an aggressive denial of the reality of risk.

Just as we as a society do not bear the full cost of the materials produced to support our experience centered culture, my father did not personally bear the full costs of his expansive life. I believe my initial chemical injury was caused by bicycle parts soaking in solvent inside the family's living space, or something similar. It was his living large, heedless of the dangers to himself and others, that laid waste to my life.

We as a society are focused on being as big as we can be, doing as much as we can, owning the nice things. My father's unspoken motto was "He who dies with the most shit, wins." From my chemical intolerance, I have learned that all of the stuff, meaning the clothing, the hobby equipment, the cars, the air in airplanes, the dry cleaning, the packaging—all of it— is toxic. Being around it causes a gradual deterioration of our health and therefore of our true selves. We are in active denial of the toxic nature of much of what we consume and experience in our quest to have big lives. Instead of being bigger in the world, trying to have more vibrant, stimulating, and experiential lives, we need to become smaller and do less to be healthy and to help our children be healthy. This is not a spiritual issue, but a practical one. We must offload products, activities, materiel, and experiences because these things are making us and our families sick.

Here is one example: Everyone wants carefree sexuality and stylish mobility, which are aspects of a life lived large. So women go on the pill and buy a new car. Modern pharmaceuticals have innocuous names, but they are powerful chemicals that affect multiple body systems. We are chemical beings, and these medications disrupt our chemical balance. Even if you don't recognize the listed potential side effects within yourself, it is a guarantee that the adverse effects to your body are on a spectrum. If the potential side effects include neurological disruption such as insomnia and depression, then the medication is making your sleep just a little worse, affecting your mood and cognition at least a little bit.

Birth control pills allow for carefree sexuality, but important studies have shown that women who take the pill are much more likely to have depression. Are birth control pills your own gateway drug, leading to sleep aids (which used to be called sleeping pills) or mood stabilizers (which used to be called antidepressants)? How can we imagine that these medications, with their complex and cumulative impacts, are not weakening us and making us more likely to need yet others for the maladies of later life?

ADHD and asthma drugs for children bring the gateway medication effect to younger lives. And why these drugs in the first place? Because of the toxins in your car and in similar indoor environments, most likely. When you open your car door, there is a smell, right? If we imagine, when we are pregnant, that this smell is not affecting the development of that tiny tender agglomeration of cells attached to our bloodstream, then we are exercising aggressive ignorance and denial in the pursuit of a consumerist fantasy. At the same time that cars and many other products have become stinkier, there has been an explosion of ADHD, asthma, and childhood cancers. There is no one minding the shop. No one is being held responsible for the damage done to the infant in the car or in your womb when you are in the car, because commercial pressures have prevented adequate testing of closed-car air quality.

There is a connection between the youthful desire for a carefree sex life and a nice car and, later on, your ill health in middle age and your child's ill health. On a practical level, if you want to be undiminished as a middle-aged person and want your child to be a whole and healthy person, you must live a smaller life. The stuff and the experiences all around us, which we are falsely told are signifiers of a large life, are making us ill in subtle ways; they are diminishing us.

When a small child is left in a hot car and dies, we ignore the obvious super-heated cloud of plastics, synthetic and coated fabrics, foams, and electronics, and blame the stupid parents for the heat exposure. Those benighted fuckers aside, we could force car manufacturers to clean up their toxi-boxes by gathering and publishing proof that the infants died from a combination of poisoning and heat, not heat alone. Remember the cloud of stench that emanates from your car on a hot day. Open your mind to the smell of your car, the chemicals oozing from your dry cleaning, and subtle aromas coming from the packaging and plastic products in your house. She who lives with the least shit, wins.

# Chapter 3 - The Mask

My mother's father was a civilian engineer supporting the US military. In the early 1940s, he was in a plane that disappeared over a remote region of Canada. He left behind a young wife who then had to go to work, as well as three girls under the age of ten: Cynthia, the oldest; my mother, Polly; and Gloria, the baby. After the loss of her husband, my grandmother became deeply reserved, maybe even cold. My mother is by nature generous and cheerful, but she also carries sadness and anger from the loss of her father when she was a child. Mom avoids confrontation and strongly denies unpleasant realities. She possesses a sort of deep feminine charisma, and people tend to automatically feel affection for her. Those close to her, such as her sisters and her children, work hard to protect her from discomfort.

My relationship with my father was fraught, and the final breach between us occurred when I was twenty-four over a box of family snapshots. At intervals over the next twenty-seven or so years, until his death, he sent me three small packets of photographs, including some random ancient negative strips, as vain attempts at reconciliation. Recently, as I reviewed what family documentation I have, looking for clues, I put these negative strips on a flatbed scanner. One image spoke to me so strongly that it was as though my father had thrown me a bone from beyond the grave.

The black-and-white photograph shows a group of five people, three adults and two children, relaxing on wide wooden steps in front of a house. They look like graduate students or young faculty outside their slightly raggedy off-campus housing. It is late summer. I recognize one adult and one child. Only the small child crawling up the steps in the middle of the frame and looking back over her shoulder is facing the camera. This small child is me at two years old. A couple of yards away, seated with her legs crossed and in profile, my mother is holding an open magazine but gazing away without purpose. She is a tall woman with graceful arms and legs and strong looking yet slender hands and feet. Her hair is pulled back in a long braid, and this accentuates her vulpine features. She is wearing a sleeveless tent-like dress that looks defiantly homemade, and she is at least six months pregnant. Next to her on the step is a drink can with graphics evocative of beer, but I can't quite read the writing and so maybe it is not alcoholic. She is twenty-eight.

Some people have different smiles for the camera than they do in real life. My mother in this snapshot has the closed-mouth, lips-only smile that was her signature. A smile can be a smokescreen to distract people from discerning one's true personality, mood, or intentions, and my mother used her smile for these purposes in photos and from day to day. The odd thing about this particular photo is that she actually seems to be suffering. There is tightness around the edges of the smile, and she looks tired, with hollow eyes. She is a young healthy woman, but she looks careworn, even haunted. I blew the image up on my computer screen and studied her face. It wasn't hard for me to imagine, and then become convinced, that this young woman had recently suffered a nasty shock. My mother, who had envisioned a certain marital and family life of happiness and joy, was struggling to reconcile her dreams with a new, brutal, and deeply unpleasant reality.

When I was almost two years old, my family was living in an apartment in Toronto. My father worked at a Canadian university and tinkered with bicycles, cars, and motorcycles. I believe my parents were happy. They had two healthy children and another on the way. Without leading disordered lives, they enjoyed the early 1960s relaxed social mores. My mother loved being pregnant and breastfeeding, and my father took many sympathetic and joyous snapshots of his family.

Then this terrible thing happened. In the Toronto apartment, there was some exposure or event, and my parents found me unresponsive and close to death (they thought). They took me to a hospital, where I stayed in a coma for several days. I was kept in the hospital for many weeks afterward. My nervous system had been badly damaged by something that my parents later told me was an unknown agent, but which I now believe they knew was a chemical exposure in our home. It can only have been terrifying for them, both the initial illness and then not knowing for about a year whether or not I would fully recover my mental faculties.

In this photograph, I see in my mother's face not only the recent horrific illness of one of her children, but much more. I see a woman in a struggle to reconcile her loyalty to her husband and her desire to maintain the marriage with the damage caused by his carelessness. I see grief over the loss of me, since she lacked the emotional and moral core to both forgive her husband and reconnect with the child she thought was going to die. Above all, I see a mask that fails to distract from her anguish, a grotesque smiley face that became her cover and her crutch for the rest of her life. In photo after photo I peer into her face, trying to make contact with the person she was, and I can't get any purchase. There is the smile but nothing behind it. As she was in real life, she is distant, a shell of a person, struggling to assemble the simulacra of a meaningful life and present herself as the whole, balanced, and loving person she wanted to be.

We all have faith that dangerous substances would not be allowed in our food, food packaging, car interior components, clothing, personal care items, mattresses, furniture, and children's toys. This is not true. For vast swaths of the items we are in close contact with every day, there is insufficient regulation, testing, or oversight. As one example, as late as 2014, Johnson & Johnson's "No More Tears" baby shampoo had formaldehyde precursors in it—"precursors" meaning chemicals that did not need to be listed on the label as formaldehyde but which chemically converted to formaldehyde immediately during use. It is cynical, and even insane, for baby shampoo to have formaldehyde in it. Scratch the surface on almost anything you touch, wear, or drive in, and it contains substances that are known neuro-disruptors, hormone disruptors, or other types of toxins.

One of the freeways by which these toxins make their way to us is through fragrance. Fragrances are insufficiently regulated. Manufacturers are not currently required to list the ingredients in fragrance, and they use known toxic agents and also untested chemicals as fragrance components. Fragrances are used as a cover for noxious smells, which are otherwise an indication that we should be careful, and also as soulless counterfeits of freshness and quality. Fragrances are used as disguises to prevent people from discerning the true nature or condition of the laundry, or the bathroom, or the chemical laden consumer product. If our laundry is not truly clean and fresh, we should allow ourselves to discern the remaining indications that the clothes aren't completely clean or completely rinsed, and then wash the clothes properly. If our bathrooms aren't truly clean, we shouldn't create a cloud of cloying toxic smell as coverup but instead should bear down and clean the bathroom thoroughly, as well as ventilate sufficiently. If you don't use air freshener in the toilet, you allow yourself to avoid the smell of poop in a natural way; whereas, if you use air freshener, you breathe in poop freely and deeply without knowing it.

I recently ordered some packets of tiny beads as a craft supply from a small online retailer. The little plastic bags had the bead descriptions handwritten on them in felt-tip pen. I smelled fragrance and contacted the seller to see where the smell was coming from. I wanted to take effective action to contain the fragrance and not allow it to make me sick, as this sort of fragrance always does. The seller said the felt-tip pen contained the fragrance. I then realized that manufacturers were using fragrance in a deeply cynical way, namely as a masking agent for smells that otherwise would alert us to danger. We and our children know to avoid certain strong chemical smells, like the smell of whiteboard markers, which once made me sick for three days. But if a cloying "fresh scented" masking fragrance is added, not only are we not alerted to the underlying ink chemicals, which are bad for us, but we also are exposed to unregulated and untested industrial fragrances, which are toxic in their own right.

Fragrance science is complex, highly advanced, and highly monetized. These substances are assembled from a surprisingly high number of ingredients, to stimulate our response at an animal level into acceptance and even enjoyment. But this is a trick played on our olfactory and neurological responses, a Trojan horse suggesting freshness and cleanliness but actually delivering toxic garbage. We as consumers and parents must purchase fragrance-free products whenever we possibly can, and we must push for our workplaces, schools, medical offices, and other environments to use only fragrance-free products.

# Chapter 4 - The True Nobility

My life feels flat. There isn't anyone I look forward to being with. There isn't anything I look forward to doing or any place I look forward to going. There isn't anything I want to accomplish.

I loved gardening, and now it leaves me uninspired. I loved birds, and now I consider a flock of hens or a pet parakeet with ennui. I enjoyed society, and now people annoy me. I wanted technical knowledge and professional success, and now these both seem pointless. I used to feel joy and exhilaration during a yoga practice, and now my daily exercise regimen is an obligation. I am going through the motions.

I long for the houses I grew up in, even though those were not happy homes. I long for my mother, my father, and my sisters, not as they were, but as I thought they were. Who was I as a child? Can I live embodied by that person rather than the disappointed and tired spirit I have become? I imagined I was self-determining and that my virtues, talents, and hard work would craft a joyous and secure life full of friends and family. I imagined I would be fit and beautiful and would contribute important ideas to the world through some yet to be chosen vocation. Unbeknownst to me, my illness was the unrecognized determinant of almost every aspect of my life. For decades I was a cripple, struggling to build a worthwhile life against fatigue, mental fogginess, chronic bad sleep, and devastating intermittent menstrual pain. I was so wrong about my life prospects that now I wonder who I am.

As a child, I made dolls, clothes for myself, and jewelry. Like a crow, I hoarded shiny or beautiful objects, whether or not they were valuable, and created small assemblages from them. I made friends with animals and smaller children. I knew I possessed attributes that signified future promise.

But instead, over four decades, my scholastic and professional accomplishments, my looks and health, and my friendships were all blasted away by illness. My career was repeatedly disrupted as I left jobs abruptly either because I was fired or on my own because I was miserable. Looking back at the person I was when I had these jobs, I now recognize the cognitive, behavioral, and mood disruptions that were the primary indicators of toxic workspaces. At the time, I would pick myself up, dust myself off, and get another job. I made friends and then alienated them through words and actions that were probably inexplicable and at the very least disconcerting and distancing. My illness caused my parents to view me with distaste, and my siblings internalized my parents' disregard. Now, in my mid-fifties, despite careful diet and regular habits, I often feel ill. My skin, hair, muscles, and connective tissues have aged in ways not explained by my treatment of them, but fully explained by a diagnosis of chronic, repeated neurological injury.

How is it possible that I kept this vision of my true self in the face of so much evidence to the contrary? I was unwilling to give up my belief in my own potential. Although I sometimes suspected that foods or environmental elements caused me trouble, the effects were varied throughout my menstrual cycle. I had terrible PMS, menstrual fatigue, and pain that were distinct from the environmental adverse effects. My husband is a private person (I'll refer to him as "Husband" from here on out) so I will not tell his story here, but he had his own chronic health problems due to chemical exposures when he was in the military. Because his were sometimes more acute and debilitating than mine, I was distracted from seeing the pattern in my own life. Neither of us received assistance from family or had independent means of support, and the area where we lived became steadily more expensive and more brutalist. As frequently happens in the Boston area, we had bad luck with neighbors—including some spectacularly poor specimens at one home of fifteen years, where a vindictive son lived next door on one side, and his dull lump of a father lived next door on the other.

If you put a frog in a pot of water and turn the stovetop on, the frog won't notice the increase in heat or hop out of the pot because the change is too gradual. This is what happened to us. As Husband and I both received professional, health, and situational setbacks, the deterioration in our lives was gradual. We didn't realize how untenable our lives had become until I became so ill at age forty-eight. Finally, using the regional real estate bubble to our advantage, we were able to leave the Boston area by selling for $750,000 the modest two-family house that we had bought for $300,000. We moved to a small town in Franklin County, Western Massachusetts. I kept my Boston-area professional job for a few more years, working exclusively from home, until I was laid off. We have no immediate money worries, and I have had a chance to finally connect the dots. With complete clarity, I see that every day my top priority must be to not be ill that day. I must stay home and make the best of it.

There are advantages to a limited life, and leisure can be a path to enlightenment. If you stay at home, you will never be in a car crash or suffer the indignities and dangers of airplanes. Reading in the news about travel disasters happening to other people will take on a special sweetness. Since you won't shop for fun, you can stop giving your friends crap presents, and you won't get any crap presents yourself. You won't get a cold or the flu.

If you stay home more, your bowels, meaning your personal fundament, will be happier. The gods among us are not the super-rich or the super-beautiful. The gods are those fortunate few who every day get out of bed, walk straight to the toilet, and drop their dirt cleanly and without strain. The true nobility are those who can drop their dirt on their own schedule, in a comfortable and private spot of their own choosing. Then, these lucky few can bathe if they want or wash their privates with a cloth, not having to exist for long periods of time with a dirty ass. This is what makes you better than other people—not money or nice clothes.

# Chapter 5 - Change in Dad

A snapshot from 1969 shows our full family, all six of us, standing outside in the sun. Dad is beaming at the camera, looking dapper and quite handsome in a nice jacket, striped tie, pressed trousers, and polished shoes. Mom is wearing a sleeveless, knee-length, dark blue silk dress with large white polka dots. The dress is fitted through the bodice and has a full and flattering skirt. She has light makeup and low, pretty heels, and she is good-looking. My sister Kirsten and I, age eight and six respectively, have on girly summer dresses and sandals. I have a plastic barrette in my hair and am holding a large plastic camera by the strap. My brother, Hunter, age four, has on a little plaid lapelled jacket that fits him perfectly, and Mom holds Amy, age two or so. The children's haircuts give them a tidy appearance. Probably we all got dressed up so that the photo could be sent to Mom's mother and Dad's parents.

Five years later, we gathered for informal family portraits on the front walkway of the house I grew up in. Mom and Dad both look as though fifteen years have gone by, not five. It is admittedly an overcast day in December, but both of them are washed-out and gray. Dad is handsome in his Brooks Brothers wardrobe, but his grin is forced, rictus style. I who know about the dental plates he needed after numerous car and bicycle accidents, can see the telltale Chiclet blocks of his fake teeth. Mom is professional with a nicely tailored jacket and a gold brooch securing a scarf around her neck. Her height as always gives her automatic elegance, but with no makeup, graying hair, and dark hollow eyes, she could be thirty-eight (her true age) or she could be fifty. The four children have bad hair, and the three youngest are wearing terrible, sad clothing. Our shoes are dirty and worn. My short-sleeved shirt is too small and weather inappropriate, my long pants are not as long as they should be, and I'm wearing bright red socks. My brother, age nine, has a haircut that must have been executed by Dad with the help of a bowl. He is inexplicably wearing a black trench coat that is much too big for him, buttoned up to his chin. Amy's clothes are the worst. At seven, she is a thin waif with an irregular haircut, wearing a strange, light blue, zippered turtleneck (which appears on me in earlier photos) and dark blue knit pants, also too short. The oldest, Kirsten, not so much, but the three youngest children look poor, like they are from a family that has been poor for a long time.

For this photo session, the primary prop is a folding lawn chair made of lightweight aluminum tubing with plastic webbing. First, Dad is sitting in it with the children behind him while Mom takes the picture. Kirsten is beside me, and her arm next to me is not around me. The hand is formed into a tight fist and is on my shoulder between us, as though she is about to punch the side of my face. Then, Kirsten is sitting in the lawn chair with Amy in her lap and the rest of us behind them, while Dad takes the picture. In this last photo, Mom has her arm around my waist, and her fingers are also curled into a fist instead of spreading out and touching my body. In possibly the only visual indication of cheer and closeness, in the second picture, Kirsten's fingers are intertwined with Amy's and the two of them look happy together. In both pictures, Hunter has both hands in the pockets of the weird trench coat, and my arms are straight down at my sides.

It is true that between 1969 and 1974 in the United States there were changes in overall standards of dress and grooming. In 1974, my mother was working and had far less time to maintain her children's wardrobes. But these pictures reflect deeper changes within our family than just wardrobe deterioration. In 1969, it mattered to my mother that she herself looked feminine and even sexy, and in 1974, it didn't. In 1969, it mattered to my parents that their children were well dressed, well coiffed, and well cared for, and in 1974, it didn't.

The mood in our house was largely determined by Dad's relative levels of contentment and frustration. I know some of the shocks and disappointments he suffered, and probably there were others that I will never know about. These blows change a person. None of us is infinitely resilient.

My brother was a sweet child who became a gentle adult with occasional outbursts of violence. My parents had done a lot of alcohol-based partying in the early years of their marriage, and my brother has personality and behavioral characteristics that perhaps suggest, just maybe, the possibility of fetal alcohol damage. My father was an observant man and would have known that, through negligence, he and Mom had damaged the cognitive abilities and brain structure of a second child, in addition to me.

Dad had two younger brothers. When I was in my late forties, I learned from my aunt Rose that both Dad and the middle boy, Rose's husband Dave, had been abused by their mother when they were small children. Rose wasn't specific, but I got the impression there were sexual aspects to the abuse. As the two boys grew older and until they started to fight back, their mother continued to use violence to control their behavior. Dave achieved professional success as an accountant but was institutionalized several times with depression and worse. He was sexual toward their two daughters and violent toward Rose, including once attempting to strangle her to death. Obviously Dave had been severely damaged by his mother, and I think my father was, too. Rose told me that when my father was around five, he did not speak for about a year, which happens sometimes when small children have been subjected to horrific abuse.

Dad's relationship with his mother was always fraught. We as a family drove to visit his parents in Detroit on a few occasions, and they visited us regularly while driving to and from Florida. I was Grandma's favorite and found her fragrant and wonderful, but she was unkind to Dad and criticized his decisions. In his thirties, he should have offloaded her but wasn't able to do it. Instead, his continued contact with her triggered distressing childhood memories of terror and helplessness.

During their fifty-year marriage, Mom and Dad grew apart and came together many times. I believe that sexual compatibility and a strong physical relationship were the pillars of their early marriage, by which I mean lots of sex. He always spoke of her with respect and deep consideration, for he craved basic kindness, which she possessed. Reflecting the intellectual milieu and with her like-minded friends, my mother embraced the self-empowering messages of 1970s feminism, including the call for fecund women to resist sexual oppression. She came under the influence of her weekly women's group and misguided messaging, such as "every rape is motivated by violence, not sex," and "a woman without a man is like a fish without a bicycle." I can imagine that my father's vigorous sexual style began to seem selfish and less sexy. She had had remarkably easy pregnancies and speedy vaginal deliveries but suffered postpartum depression after Amy's birth. Probably after four children, as she inserted her diaphragm to prepare for intercourse with her husband, she was dismayed by the changes in her bodily sexual apparatus and what these changes said about her wifely identity. She stopped wanting to have sex with him. I know this because, even though it was none of my business, I saw that the tube of spermicidal jelly stored with her diaphragm in an open basket on her dresser stayed in the same half-used shape for years.

This was a profound change in their lives. I'm guessing my father had a strong sexual nature from the frequent sexual jokes and references he made, even around his children. As his opportunity for the regular expulsion of semen into a woman stopped, he became clogged up with rage-inducing jism. Men want to make war and blow things up when they aren't fucking regularly. This is a human truth. Dad had extramarital sex and I'm not judging, as I imagine for him it was a bodily necessity. However pleasurable and exciting these outside relationships must have been, I'm sure they were also stressful and a source of guilt. Due to pragmatic imperatives, this outside sex would only have been occasional compared to the regular sex that had previously been available within his marriage.

Dad received tenure and taught for many years at the university. He worked hard to deliver quality instruction to his students, and his books demonstrate both heavy research and thoughtful, relevant analysis. But he never fit in at his job. Both he and I had in-your-face arrogance when it came to our native intelligence. Just as I did in high school and at my professional jobs, my father wished to be adored and celebrated for his raw talent and accomplishments by the same people he triumphed over and despised as inferior. Not surprisingly, neither of us got our wish. Despite job security, considerable free time and schedule flexibility, and university support for his numerous sabbaticals and extensive travel, he wasn't content at work. He complained bitterly about his colleagues and did not make good friends.

However it happened, my father's faith in the basic goodness of the world and people, that we are all born with and that we cling to ferociously, became irrevocably damaged. What had earlier been charisma, enthusiasm, desire to connect with others, and a predominant cheerfulness became insularity, eccentricity, and a distrust of the motivations of other people. He developed a bad temper and became intolerant of noise in the house. He often seemed uncomfortable in his own skin and vaguely agitated, and he frequently talked about his own feelings in a way that was self-pitying and unedifying. As my father lost faith in the ability of the world to provide everything he wanted, he turned inward for comfort and support. He pampered himself with private luxuries, toys, and pleasures. He did not have the outward generosity to support his children as they grew out of infancy, and, aware of this failure, he resented them for their reasonable demands for clothing, proper nutrition, attention, and guidance.

My father became obsessed with money. In the early 1970s when Mom wanted her own checking account as a feminist gesture, he readily agreed. The bifurcation of family liquid cash allowed him to fulfill a cherished dream—to save his own money. In her generous and easygoing way, Mom paid for most family incidentals like food and clothing, and Dad established a mailing address and locked file drawers in his university office for the records of his secret hoarded assets. His favorite domestic evening pastime became sitting in a comfortable corner in gentle yellow-tinted light, still replete from a large and tasty lunch, clothed in well-cut natural fibers and doodling columns of figures representing schemes for wealth accumulation, while his ill-clothed, undernourished, and ignorant children tiptoed around him.

# Chapter 6 - Domestic Violence

My patient and tolerant mother would occasionally become so provoked that she hit us, even when in public places, in a way that would have gotten her hauled before the tribunal today. Fifty years ago, what was called spanking was widely accepted. Children do need to be controlled and punished sometimes—I get that. I also get that Dad grew up with violence, not only in his home but also in his working-class Detroit neighborhood when he was a teenager and on ships and in ports around the world when he was a merchant marine as a young man. He had been in many fights and had been beaten up, sometimes badly. I get that he was accustomed to hitting and beating—the pounding of hands or fists against someone else's skin, muscle, bone. But how can a powerfully built and athletic grown man hit, and I mean hit hard, a child of seven? This was different from spanking. I try to find common ground with my father, and this is one of the areas I come up short. I remember him starting toward me, knowing he was going to hit me, and me shaking and screaming in terror. He didn't have these wells of rage and frustration in the early years of our family.

Probably what many of the beatings were about, and he didn't even know this himself, was noise in the house. We weren't bad, but we were children, and there were four of us. Naturally we talked to each other and moved around, and this movement made some noise. My father wanted to dampen the natural exuberance of his children; his neurology and psyche were damaged and not resilient to stimulation because he had himself suffered abuse as a child. But children don't creep around like mice. Why have so many children if you can't bear to hear them?

Dad became unsettled when family members focused on something other than himself. He enjoyed the intense feelings that came from making emotional connections, especially if he was in control. In the evenings or on weekends, he would sit by himself, alternately listening to creaking and chitchat from our rooms and pleasuring himself by making money-doodles and counting his piles of gold. Occasionally a child would raise his or her voice a little bit or drop something, and he would fidget and clench his teeth. After a slightly louder noise, he would blow up and chase us down throughout the house. At the time, the rage and violence seemed to be triggered by our simple existence. He beat me repeatedly for what he called "arrogance," which label I tried and failed to connect to anything I had said or done.

Kirsten was Mom's favorite. She was not hit as much, and neither was tiny Amy. There wasn't physical violence toward Mom, but I allow for the possibility that she was passive when he beat us because she had been cowed by emotional or verbal pressure during the early years of their marriage.

He hit us, he yelled at us with rage in his voice, and he terrorized us through threats of violence. This ended for me around the time I grew breasts, but even for the next few years I was apprehensive that he didn't know it was time for him to stop. I last saw my father when I was in my mid-twenties, but well into my forties I had elaborate and full-color dreams about him stalking me and doing me violence. He was a scary dude—not 100 percent of the time, but a lot of the time.

Mom did not visibly object. Did she sense that the beatings provided him with intense physical contact that was a substitute for the missing contact between the two of them? With limited access to my parents' inner lives, I can only guess the reasons for Dad's general awfulness during those years. Mom would know for sure which of his demons was chewing out his guts back then. She chose him over us, in defiance of commonsense fairness and her psychological training and in order not to be alone.

I get that sometimes parents become so frustrated that they lash out and spank or yell at their children—even children they love and wish to be happy in the world. But now I see that this chronic and explosive violence was a sign of Dad's inability to wish me well. With this new understanding of the beatings, I must now reinterpret Dad's other actions, which previously I either excused as eccentricity or conveniently ignored and then forgot. Mom is considered by everyone she knows to be kind-hearted and gener- ous, a skilled psychotherapist, but since she tolerated the beatings I must now reexamine her character and emotional capabilities as well. My parents are accomplished people with obvious virtues. I hear the voices of my parents' neighbors, colleagues, and friends calling me an ungrateful child, saying of course my parents loved me and that my mother is a saint. I hear my siblings denying the beatings were so severe and calling me self-indulgent and wrong- minded. I naturally want to suppress the shame of the beatings. The belief that the world is basically good goes hand in hand with the belief that your mother loves you; do I have to relinquish my faith in both of these consolations?

For my whole life until now, I believed that my par- ents loved me and that their flaws and our family's dynamics prevented them from fully expressing that love. Now I must make a choice. I can see myself with extreme clarity as a tender lump of exposed flesh in a dangerous world, susceptible to environmental toxins that rip apart my mental equilibrium and that could destroy every one of my days during the brief time I have left upon this earth. Or, I can continue to embrace the false but comforting beliefs that have caused me to spend decades in an impaired and struggling condition. I am a courageous and determined person, and I absolutely claim the truth of my own history. It doesn't matter what other people think. This is not a nostalgic exercise but a practical imperative. The current chemical- and fragrance-laden world is poisonous to me. I must learn if my parents watched me struggle with neurological impairment while fully aware of its true cause so that I can summon the strength and conviction to just stay home and implement nonconventional approaches to the mechanics of everyday life. With incremental days spent not ill, perhaps I can claw back some measure of health and joy.

# Chapter 7 - Travel

In the 1960s and 1970s, there had not yet been the explosion of chemicals and fragrances in consumer products, and my parents didn't buy standard consumer products anyway. Our homes and the schools I attended were built of wood and real plaster and not air-conditioned and neither were our cars air-conditioned, so mostly I was in spaces with good air circulation and good air quality. Despite these healthy environments, as a girl I had symptoms of nervous system damage. I struggled to find my voice at school and in social situations. Now I know this apparent shyness was a continuing symptom of my initial neurological injury.

Because of my reading and writing skills, my parents put me in the first grade as I was just turning five. So, I was about two years younger and much smaller than my classmates. Although I was well-coordinated and determined, I was unable to catch a ball or frisbee, kick a ball, or hit anything with a racket or bat, so I failed at group sports. Instead, I perfected the cartwheel and invented balancing postures on my bike, like standing on the seat, or riding with one foot on a pedal and the other leg high up in the air with the bike leaning away as counterbalance. I rode my father's full-size bike by pedaling through the center below the crossbar.

By the time I was ten and in the sixth grade, I shamelessly grubbed for money every way I could. I developed a babysitting clientele and filled in on an afternoon paper route. From Mom, I got a penny for every ten weeds pulled in the garden and a penny for every four snails or slugs collected and killed. I proofread Dad's books and got a dollar for every typographical or grammatical error I found. I tried to sell greeting cards that I bought through an ad in the back of a comic book. I tried to sell bead jewelry that I made. With my earned savings, I bought a new adult-sized three-speed bicycle that I chose myself, planning to suffer a little inconvenience from it being too big so that it would fit me for many years afterward. A couple of years later, I bought myself a sewing machine.

Dad researched his books in the great libraries in big cities, and for longer stays we went with him. We spent a summer in California in a house next to an apricot orchard. For the road trips to and from, Mom and Dad turned the back of our station wagon into an enormous platform bed for lounging, eating, and sleeping. Once when Dad was driving, Mom was napping in the rear, the other children were scattered here and there, and I was leaning against the back hatch, holding a book with one hand and picking my nose with the other. Eyes still glued to the book and with an enormous half-dry half-wet booger on one finger, I wormed the booger-laden finger around in the debris field in the back of the car, found a suitable resting spot based on feel, and scraped my finger back and forth. I thought I was alone, so to speak, but then I heard my mother objecting mildly from way up near the front, "That's my toe."

The family spent a summer in New York City, which then was much filthier than it is now. The newspapers were filled with coverage of a recent stabbing death in an area of Central Park near our apartment, and I looked for dried pools of blood whenever we entered the park. Amy, almost five and already a secretive and acquisitive creature, devoted herself to eating the discarded chewing gum she found all over the city. Well, not exactly eat. She was old enough to understand the basic principle of gum. She would swap gum in her mouth for other gum throughout the day. By unhappy coincidence, when adults offload gum, they do it at the eye level of a small child. We'd be walking along with Mom, getting to know the city, and, if one of us looked back, there she would be, scrabbling her dirty, worn fingernails against a subway entrance railing or underneath a park bench. She had a ruminative focus most of that summer as she continually discovered, tasted, and then left behind these tailings of humanity. It seemed to me that she was trying to ingest into her tiny white body the dirtiest and most dangerous part of that very dirty and dangerous city. I remember thinking, "Who *does* that?" But it was Amy who got to know the city and its people best, while the rest of us limited ourselves to looking at shops and buildings.

During my seventh-grade year, we lived in Bonn, Germany, with the support of a Fulbright fellowship Dad got. We children went to German schools. Mine was new construction. Kirsten and I took the city streetcars by ourselves to school and to visit with classmates. In piecing together the history of my illness, this is the first instance I can remember where a specific environment triggered a long-term manifestation of neurological symptoms. I loved learning, and the excellent German educational system taught Latin, Greek, French, business, and physics, as well as lots of math, which I especially loved. I remember not feeling well generally, struggling to stay awake in school, and also struggling to learn, which was unusual for me.

The following summer the family traveled extensively in Europe, the six of us and our luggage squeezed into Dad's

European car of choice, a Volkswagen Beetle. We children learned to eat, sleep, and pee when we had the chance and also to carry our own city maps and know how to use them. We understood at a cellular level that if we lost something, or stumbled, or got separated from the rest of the family, it was our own fault. Dad took us to museums and even into antique shops full of fragile items because we were trained to hold our hands together behind our backs the entire time we were inside these places.

One of our trips was to Italy, and it included visiting the Roman ruins of Pompeii near Naples. Dad drew me aside to show me an ancient wall fresco of a naked man with an erect penis the size of an arm, with the penis resting on a scale. "Worth its weight in gold," Dad said, leering at me. I giggled as a cover for discomfiture and shrugged this episode off as just Dad being weird. In Florence, Kirsten, then thirteen, took Hunter and me across the river to the non-touristy side for a long exploratory walk for the day. We inadvertently picked up a grown man like other folks might a stray dog. This man followed us silently at a distance for hours until we passed back over the river to meet up with our parents late in the afternoon. My intrepid sister knew how to herd her younger siblings around a strange city and order a cheap lunch in a foreign language, but not how to shake an adult stalker.

When I came back to the United States to a new school for the eighth grade, I was quiet and had trouble making friends. Toxic building materials in the newly constructed school I attended in Germany had reinjured my nervous system, and during the following years my cognition and behavior were still affected. I was pretty and made good grades but had trouble fitting in. There were social cliques made up of the children of academics, which I should have been a part of, but I didn't manage to integrate into these groups.

My parents' lifestyle didn't alleviate my social awkwardness. We children were not allowed to watch television, read comic books, or listen to popular music because Dad insisted that popular culture was destructive garbage. We were not allowed to eat candy. Except for certain arrangements between my mother and Kirsten, my parents would not pay for lessons or take us to birthday parties or other social or after-school events. This had a silver lining because their cars were embarrassing. I almost never had new or sufficient clothing and was usually ashamed of my appearance. We did understand that because Mom worked she didn't have time to drive us around town and take us shopping, and we were fiercely proud of her for working. Our friends were not welcome in the house because of Dad's low tolerance for alien activity or noise, but we children could go anywhere as long as we were home for dinner at five o'clock. Like a small pack of feral dogs getting on with life in spite of dirt and hunger, we explored empty lots, railroad tracks, and backyards.

Dad said that, instead of buying things, our family traveled and read books. I agreed with him that our family was better than everyone else, and I admired my parents for consciously rejecting consumerist junk. I'm glad now that instead of watching television, I scrounged up gainful employment at an early age and bought my own tools and transportation. Throughout my life, I never had trouble getting a job or accepting even supposedly degrading forms of employment. While many of their lifestyle choices were motivated by Dad's desire to save money and preserve his own free time, I'm proud of my parents for not allowing cultural garbage into our home. My family's nonconforming lifestyle helped prepare me for the difficult transition I needed to make when I was forty-eight.

At forty-eight, when I was made so ill from my job, it was by far the worst chemical reinjury of my life. In addition to the neurological distress caused by the primary exposure within the workspace, I acquired a secondary and permanent sensitivity to many common chemicals. As I slowly recovered over the next seven or so years (which process continues as of the writing of this book), I examined the possessions and habits of my life and questioned many of them. I did not need to wear certain clothes, buy shoes, buy kitchen gadgets, or eat the fashionable ingredients. I didn't need to read books or magazines, listen to NPR's *All Things Considered*, know who Frank Gehry is, or be familiar with the latest spoutings of Gloria Steinem. I didn't need to save money or invest in mutual funds or stocks. I did not need to wear lipstick, shave my legs, dye the gray out of my hair, bathe every day, clean my house and tidy the yard to a certain standard, or keep the house a certain temperature. I didn't even need to maintain relationships with problematic people such as family members. Everything was up for renegotiation.

My so-called illness is actually a form of enlightenment. Through my struggles, I have learned terrible yet crucial truths. These chemicals have an exaggerated effect on me, but they are harmful to everyone. We as a society don't have tests for determining proper threshold exposures to the many industrial and consumer chemicals that are introduced every year, nor have we even developed tools to detect when these harmful substances are present in our lives. In lieu of government sanctioned testing and detection of harmful chemicals and good-faith cooperation by industry, I offer my suffering to the world. I am a prophet whose teachings can help you protect yourself and your loved ones.

Start small, by airing out your car before you put your children into it, purchasing nonfragranced laundry products, and not allowing any stinky printed material like newspapers or junk mail into your house. Then when you are ready, consider these next steps:

1. Find alternatives to fragranced and heavily chemicalized body care and cleaning products. Artificial fragrances contain chemicals that are known neuro-disruptors. If you limit your exposure to these compounds, you will sleep better.

2. Do not purchase clothes that must be dry-cleaned. Find other things to wear. Do not store dry-cleaned items in your living space. If you must dry-clean something, air it out without its plastic before bringing it into the house.

3. Pay attention to consumer products that have a smell, like books and magazines, packaging, and plastic items. Many soft plastic things are made in molds. The mold-release compounds have a sickly sweet smell that you can wash off, if you must bring these items into your house.

4. Pay attention to the smell of cloth consumer goods, like sheets and clothing. Much imported cloth is routinely treated with pesticides, and probably your child's new clothes smell "nice" because a masking fragrance has been used to cover up processing and manufacturing residues, as well as pesticides.

5. Bring as little mail as possible into your house. Find a place to air out any necessary individual sheets of paper, and dump all extraneous mail components into an outside bin.

6. Pay more attention to the smell of your car, and let plenty of air in while driving. Some indoor car chemicals are strongest when the car is new, and others develop over time as the interior plastic components degrade with age. Consider your car to be, not a symbol of freedom, but a toxic box to which you should limit your family's exposure. Before buying a new car, research "less toxic cars."

7. Do not buy things or paint the nursery for a new baby. Try to see clearly every item and surface in that room. It turns out that humans have an excellent sense of smell; especially in the nursery, pay attention to what the smells are telling you.

Thoughtful people are working on this problem, and there is an ever-increasing number of websites offering guidance and product suggestions. I have listed a few of them in the appendix. Protect yourself and your family, and also please consider becoming a voice for change within your community.

∞

Make no mistake about it: when you choose to dye your hair, wear dry-cleaned clothes, buy a stack of magazines, or purchase a new car, you are mortgaging the health of your children, both born and unborn. This is not a theoretical impact. We already know that our consumption is contributing indirectly to overall worldwide health through environmental damage, but we may not know that it is having a direct impact on ourselves and our families. Erroneous and faith-based assumptions that the government is looking out for us and wouldn't allow harmful substances in consumer products, that large American corporations would only distribute safe products, or that we as Americans are protected from underregulated imported products and food are preventing us from seeing our world clearly.

# Chapter 8 - Beauty and the Secret Society

⁓

The eye is drawn to the attractive person in any group, and anyone looking at our family pictures looks first at me. Most women feel unsettled when they meet me and most men are attracted, although I have no interest in the volume of sex on offer based on my current beauty. The pressure to be beautiful is a trap, I'm thinking, and it is better to not attract attention. I dress as badly as I can without incurring public disapprobation, cut my own hair, keep my mustache, bathe not often, and use no beauty products, and it is often after noon when I clean my teeth for the first time in a day. Yet all day long my husband, age seventy-four, feels an interest in intimacy (how else can I put this) when he looks at me. What this tells me is that he loves me, yes, but also that if you are naked or even just nearby, beauty routines are unnecessary given the innate enthusiasm of most men and the inherent yumminess of most women.

My mother was tall with high cheekbones, thick hair, lovely skin, and thin ankles. For her work as a PhD psychologist, she had a no-frills grooming and wardrobe formula. She wore colorful lipstick and a hint of mascara, a simple blouse with blazer and scarf, an A-line skirt, nylon hosiery, and low-heeled pumps. She looked just fine all of the time and elegant a lot of the time. She was matter-of-fact about her own nudity within the household, so if she was getting dressed at home or while we were traveling, we children had plenty of chances to see her breasts. She took to heart the 1970s feminist messaging about burning bras and also didn't care about her nipples showing through her clothing, which they did. Her boobs are burned into my brain as strongly as her face, and I found both to be exceptionally beautiful. Well into adulthood, in photographs or mirror views where my breasts looked more like my memory of my mother's breasts, I liked my breasts, and when my breasts looked less like hers, I didn't like them so much.

My older sister, Kirsten, was lovely as a small child, with enormous eyes that were kaleidoscopes of hazel and green, slender limbs, and fine-boned features. Then her teeth became too large in her face, required many years of orthodontia, and ended up straight but protruding such that she needed to stretch her lips to cover them. A front tooth died, and its mismatched replacement had a disconcerting dark base. She was not naturally graceful. In photographs, she tried to compensate for lack of effortless beauty by smiling broadly, often with her head thrown back, a gesture she didn't use in real life. All you see is mouth. She was chunky in a way that doctors and fair-minded people would never call overweight, but she had a little layer of fat around her middle, and I'm sure that while seated in summer shorts, she looked down at her pale flattened upper-thigh meat with dismay. I admit unkindness, but I am grateful my breasts didn't look like hers.

And there's more. As a preteen and teenager, Kirsten frequently developed inflamed pustules in her eyelash pores. As in,

"She got a stye in her eye." No one else in the family got them, so probably she scratched her own ass-crack and then rubbed her eyes or had some other unhygienic habit the way children do. Whatever the unsavory cause, these styes repeatedly gave her temporary partial blindness and disfigurement. Logically, I'm aware there is no causal connection between one's tendency to kindness and the gift of physical beauty, but because Kirsten used to hit and pinch me and then look for the bruises, for me her appearance always reflected her inner self. Once I was at the top of a steep driveway about to ride down it on my bike. Ignoring my protestations and with a little knowing smile, Kirsten shoved me down the slope under the guise of helping me get started. I landed on my face and one knee, required surgery to stitch my upper lip together, had a lopsided smile for the next two decades, and can still see the scar on my knee. Another time she begged for a bite of the sandwich I was holding and then lurched her mouth forward like one of Sigourney Weaver's aliens, biting my finger badly. Then she laughed. She wasn't reprimanded for either of these events or for others. After I turned eight or so, almost certainly for my safety and to my parents' credit, our sleeping quarters were always in separate rooms. Even now I smile at the memory of her styes—sweets for the sweet.

Also when I was eight or so, my mother shed grooming rituals and sexual signifiers. Her chestnut hair, which used to fall to her waist in the thickest, lushest braid you've ever seen, was cut to a no-nonsense chin-length bob and allowed to gray naturally. Her buttocks and thighs became large, disproportionate to her waist and upper body. Mom stopped shaving her legs, which then became thick with long curly dark hair. I mean, shockingly hairy, like a hairy man. She stopped wearing a bra completely, even when jogging or running errands in a T-shirt, and didn't buy new underwear. She cleaned up and looked professional for her job, with a blazer concealing her nipples and nylon hose flattening and obscuring the wiry leg hair, but her leisure wardrobe was disreputable and showed she didn't care anymore.

Mom and Kirsten started to share secrets. I know this because Kirsten had knowledge about other people she could not have discovered on her own and because Kirsten started to channel Mom with respect to other family members. She knew whether or not particular friends of our parents had a happy marriage, she expressed mature empathy toward something inappropriate Dad said or did, or she looked out for the two youngest children in a way that suggested filial concern. She became more self-assured in her affect, even smug, and her understanding of the world was inexplicably far beyond her calendar age. She was never teasing or coy about either the source of her new power or what else she knew—both were nonnegotiable.

I remember being with the two of them and sensing a force field between them. They didn't speak to each other in front of other people, they observed and judged people with a shared understanding, and they were often out and about alone together. Sometimes a piece of jewelry or clothing would appear in the household that they both used, while other family members had no idea where it had come from. Or, Kirsten would inexplicably receive an advantage that the other children never got, like a ride in Mom's car, a haircut, or lunch with Mom and her friends, and these events were not discussed or justified. Kirsten dressed far better than I did, and the mechanics underlying her wardrobe acquisitions were shrouded in mystery. I used to think Mom could have done better; she could have picked me instead, who was smarter, prettier, and nicer.

When I was thirteen and in the ninth grade, I liked a boy named Richard and he liked me. He was tall and outgoing, with big brown eyes, and I had the chaste hots for him. He was fantastic, and I wish I could go back in time and scoop him up. One day Mom, Kirsten, and I were hanging out in the living room, and I was going on about how handsome, athletic and smart he was. I said I would name my favorite houseplant after Richard, and I held the plant in my lap and caressed the central shaft that held an unfurled leaf. After a pause in which Kirsten looked at me coldly, she said emphatically, "Why don't you just *fuck* it?" and Mom chimed in, "Yeah, really." I felt like an idiot for stroking the pointy shape of the houseplant while invoking my boyfriend's name, but the leaf wasn't shaped like a penis, and my impulses were innocent. They were not sexual but were instead the natural tendency of an imaginative child to name an object after an adored person. I found the plant beautiful and felt close to it, and I found Richard beautiful and felt close to him. It sounds odd, but it wasn't. Mom and Kirsten could have chosen to excuse my childish enthusiasm and awkwardness, but they saw someone who had the capacity and opportunity for love and sex, compared to their own lack of sexual love. They were bitter. Instead of displaying generosity and understanding, they took the chance to recast my words as perverse and obnoxious.

Their response at that time was typical. When they looked at me, they felt fat, unsexy, and unlovable. This happened so often and made them feel so bad that they imagined I intended to hurt them. They treated me as if I was vaguely malevolent and my sexuality was destructive. Now I see that for decades, both of these women whom I loved and whose affection I desperately wanted, regarded me as an injurious force in their lives. Even as I blindly assumed that Mom and Kirsten reciprocated my love for them, they found common ground in objecting to what I did or said. Both needed to believe in their own virtues so their words and actions were subtle, but together they maintained a steady and long-lived belief in my despicability.

Here is where the story becomes scary. When a mother colludes with one daughter to create an alternate persona for a second daughter who is innocent, then the mother is going down a dark path that will lead to self-harm. Now I see that Mom did struggle with discomfort when the two of us were together and that she avoided contact with me because it hurt. When I was thirteen, I explained away Mom's discomfiture as being caused by Dad admiring my academic achievements and finding Kirsten's to be deficient, but I was in denial. There was far more going on.

It is wonderful to make a dog love you and also make that dog dislike someone you dislike, but Kirsten was more complicated than a dog. While the secrets made Kirsten feel special and better than other children, this messaging wasn't borne out by her experience in the real world, meaning boys, popular girls, the mirror. Dad was unapologetic about liking pretty people best, and he didn't manage to be kind to her about her looks or her achievements. As Kirsten grew up, she struggled to create a positive affirming self-identity and tended to attribute to other people harmful intentions that did not exist. Both Mom and Kirsten knew that whatever the immediate consolations, their collusion in smearing me was based on a destructive lie. This shaped the people they were for the rest of their lives.

Although I don't find Kirsten likable anymore, I don't blame her for treating me the way she did. She was not the initiator, and this dynamic started so early that she didn't have a choice. She could not have been expected to refuse membership in their secret society, in which the rewards were unconditional intimacy and adult wisdom. All she had to do was choose Mom over me, the middle daughter. To have your mother's unconditional love is an enormous gift, perhaps the biggest one that a human can receive, and Mom was generous to Kirsten not only with information and affection but also with clothes, cash, credit, travel, meals out, and other goodies. Over the years and in ways not consciously acknowledged, Kirsten sacrificed any chance of a true relationship with me in favor of lifelong intangible and tangible largesse from Mom.

To their conscious minds I was a shitty little show-off, and to their subconscious minds I was a source of pain. I was oblivious to their feelings. From childhood on, I gobbled a steady diet of English-language classic novels. Just like Hollywood movies, these stories base their resolution on the ideal of virtue rewarded. I developed a firm faith that the basic kindliness of people and organizations would reward a hardworking, handsome, and intelligent person such as myself with love and a happy life. If I did suffer adversity or misfortune, the world would rally to my support because the world was basically good. Now I know life doesn't work this way. No one is looking out for us. Loss, illness, and death come to us regardless of our natural gifts and in most instances regardless of our behavior. The only thing you can do is develop practical approaches to limiting and managing your losses before you die.

Embrace the reality of your body. Few women have perky breasts. If you wear them low, you can gather unto yourself the power of this truth. Instead of propping them up and harboring secret shame about droop, take comfort in these gentle and delicious sacks of fat. Let the girls jostle gently and healthily about, and don't press them for long hours into synthetic foam constructions that exude chemical residues (right next to lymph node central!). To expect adult breasts to stand at attention is not reasonable. Breasts are scrumptious and everyone loves them, wherever they are resting. Just find ways to keep the nipples under wraps because it is not possible for man, woman, or child to resist staring at a nipple, any nipple.

Let your hair go gray and do not get plastic surgery or similar face-plumping or face-freezing treatments. Hair dyes are bad for you and your children, born and unborn. More studies are proving what is commonsensically obvious, namely that artificial adjustments to your appearance cause emotional distance. You become less human. You may think you are more attractive, but you are repellant and untrustworthy at a subliminal level.

Instead of push-up bras and Botox, stay home as much as you can while wearing pajama-like clothing. Get in the habit of initiating cuddles during which your mature and naturally fragrant yummies are pressing against your loved one with thin fabric or none between you. That should do the trick.

# Chapter 9 - Typical Day

Yesterday, I went out with a friend to have fun. While in his car, I held my half-face cartridge respirator up to my face almost the entire time, but I neglected to crack the car window. We went to a local stone quarry to look at slabs of schist and dream of garden accents; then to lunch in our favorite restaurant in the beautiful village of Shelburne Falls, Massachusetts; then to an ephemera shop; and later an artists' cooperative. After eating I held the mask to my face for the rest of our time in the restaurant, and I also wore it in the artists' cooperative. We admired the town vistas and chatted comfortably. I remember feeling youthful, attractive, and optimistic in the restaurant as I outlined the next steps for several of my projects.

In the car ride back to our hometown, I had trouble finding words. Normally he and I have long upbeat conversations, but yesterday, at the end of our outing, I started using a bossy tone when he was discussing a decision he needed to make. Recognizing the symptoms of chemical exposure, I forced myself to be silent so I wouldn't accidentally say anything strange or hurtful. I normally use curse words sparingly in conversation, but when I have an adverse exposure, foul language wants to come out of me along with negative comments generally. I was careful to be quiet until he dropped me at home. For the rest of the day I was unmotivated. I did food preparation with such a lack of finesse that the next day the questionable concoction went into a compost bin. I sat doing handwork and watching a mystery series on the computer. In the evening, I abused a zit on my neck while taking note of a wan and aged face. I went to bed at nine thirty and had stupid dreams alternating with unhappy wakefulness before waking up for good at three thirty in the morning.

Today, midmorning the day after our outing, I am groggy and ill, as if I am hungover. I have a tiny headache, no ideas, and find any stimulation to be annoying. My muscles are achy. The problem is that, despite my mask, I had ingested the vapors of the off-gassing plastics and other components in my friend's car interior. I wasn't careful enough when alternately talking to him and breathing through the mask and did not introduce enough fresh air into the car as we were driving along. The effects were cumulative. By the end of the outing, I was struggling. Because my nervous system has been damaged by prior chemical exposures, I don't have the toxin-fighting mechanisms that normal people do. This tiny amount of ingested poisons enters my system without barriers and has a significant effect on my mood, cognition, and behavior.

Yesterday's exposure and its results were mild. Today, I am still able to carry on a conversation, perform household tasks, brush my teeth, and even haltingly type up this description of events. But I have been diminished and feel worn out. There is nothing I want to accomplish, and nothing I am looking forward to.

To help me manage my illness, I have a paper grid containing, for each calendar day, a checklist of all of the activities I should be doing in my life. There are about forty items, in categories like hygiene, housework, handwork, projects, and wellness. I try to check off about ten items every day. When I have been chemically poisoned, I clutch this piece of paper and search for something brainless I still can accomplish. The standard for earning a checkmark is generous. If I shuffle-jog around the block, picking up a *Game of Thrones* DVD set at the library and some cash at the bank, that counts as two check-marks: "walk/run" and "household errands." I'm able to propel myself forward in a slightly brain-dead, tired state, drawing a veil over how crappy I feel. Fake it till you make it.

When we were kids, the family ate dinner at the same time every day. Dad liked being the center of attention. Using grunts and facial expressions to make threats of aggression, he monitored the allocation of food, especially any small amount of meat that had been prepared. He liked to talk about people in the neighborhood or at his job and his own accomplishments. These meals were a comfort because the family was together and I loved being with them, but Dad was frequently in a bad mood and sometimes he would just blow up with rage. The remainder of that meal would be spent in silence until one of us children was brave enough to say the required, "May I please be excused?"—meaning, *get me the fuck out of here.*

Instead of a handbag, Mom carried a capacious open-style briefcase, almost a portable office, for the papers and personal effects she needed during her business day. Her large zippered wallet, overstuffed with receipts, photographs, promotional cards, and paper cash, hung out in her briefcase, along with cans of Tab diet drink, pens, mail, files, keys, stamps, basic makeup, and various other possessions. She had an endearing habit. She paid for everything with paper money and then tossed all coins received as change into the briefcase. It would become heavier and heavier with the puddle of coins at the bottom. I monitored the puddle, and once every couple of years she let me dump everything out and gather the coins into paper tubes for her to exchange at the bank.

Amy, hungry but too young to work for money, started taking coins from the bottom of Mom's briefcase to buy sandwiches, desserts, and candy in the local restaurant and shop district a short walk away. I knew this because, at the same time that the puddle became more pennies than quarters, a friend told me she saw Amy, age eight or so, sitting by herself in an upscale café eating a piece of chocolate cake. I figured that cake cost about $4, a vast sum of money at the time. There were also wrappers from expensive European chocolates under her bed. I was impressed by my sister's style. When I mentioned the evidence of theft to Mom, it was clear she already knew about it. Probably she accepted the practice since Amy needed the nutrition. It was a way for the two of them to communicate, meaning Amy had initiated a back channel for emotional connection that Mom hadn't otherwise managed. Amy graduated to small bills and then to larger bills, and Mom finally summoned the courage to say something when she was no longer able to ignore the rate of disappearing twenties.

We admired our father for researching and writing books. I thought he had achieved immortality and greatness by being published repeatedly. In his early books, I who know him well see someone who is reaching for the truth and trying to make sense of important human stories. But then he changed, and his later books are weaker. In his choice of words and the nature of his observations, I see someone who is struggling and whose self-referential bias is preventing him from viewing people with generosity or the world with clarity.

When I was thirteen, at the time Dad was buying bronze sculptures in the auction houses in Europe, Kirsten and I stayed with him for several weeks in his apartment in Germany. The three of us drove to Paris in Dad's Beetle for a few days as tourists. We stayed in a cheap hotel, and one evening Dad opened a can of sauerkraut and ate part of it. He left the can on the floor in such a way that when I got up to go to the toilet, I sliced my big toe open on the lid. I had to spend the night lying still on my back and with my leg elevated on a chair to staunch the bleeding and avoid a trip to a doctor for stitches. The next day he became agitated when we were in terrible Paris traffic and, while exiting the car to get directions, he slammed his thumb in the car door. I was surprised that a thumb could fit in a closed car door for any length of time, but somehow it did fit there until he managed to open the door with his other hand. Kirsten and I thought this was hysterically funny. While we tried not to laugh from inside the car, he hopped around outside of it, shaking his injured hand and cursing.

As each of us in turn entered adolescence, Dad separated us from the pack for tortured conversations that must have served for him as talk therapy. He preferred the Waffle House, where customers could park for a long time in comfortable booths without pressure to spend more money, and where the waitresses called him "sweetheart" and refilled his coffee for free. I remember him complaining bitterly about Mom's inability to discipline the children, telling me Amy was a thief and a liar, complaining about his job and colleagues, and boasting about the money he was making on his various schemes. He frequently spoke of his terror of dying alone and in a deteriorated state, as he said, "in the blood and the shit and the piss." But once, during his upsetting and narcissistic ramblings, I did learn something important.

The two of us were in a booth at the Waffle House, and Dad was ranting about Mom's money—not the coins sloshing around in her briefcase, but money he calculated she must have been earning from her work. "Where does Polly put it?" he said about twenty times like a mantra, while pockets of foam gathered in the corners of his mouth. From his theatrical posturing and grimacing as he attempted to project wounded virtue, I intuited it was actually he who was hiding assets. Finally he paused, and I saw my chance to ask him something that had been bothering me. I said I knew Mom always had a lot going on, but that she didn't seem to connect with me. By my tone, facial expression, and choice of words, I soft-pedaled to get a bit of insight rather than risk alarming him into silence. He said, and these were his words (almost exactly, if not exactly): that something had happened when I was small, that she had always blamed him for, and that prevented her from ever feeling close to me. I stored his words away for later, sensing they were important even if I had no context for them then.

This partial and vague admission of responsibility is the smoking gun for my chemical injury during infancy and my lifelong ill health. More than forty years later and in the context of my desperate efforts to solve the two central mysteries of my life, this tidbit of conversation, meaningless at the time, is a priceless treasure. Why was I ill so often? Why did my mother not like me? These two questions have the same answer. While sitting with me in that restaurant booth, whatever his inner demons and despite the tizzy he had worked himself into, my father reached for the truth when I asked him to.

# Chapter 10 - Journal

As I look over the sweep of my time so far, the years when I was fourteen and fifteen seem vibrant, full of color and meaning. This was when I was the true expression of myself. Afterward, I tried to patch my life together as pieces kept falling apart, including my relationships with loved ones, my jobs, my health, Husband's health, and my living arrangements. For a couple of years I was lucky, and then I was unlucky.

I kept a journal back then. When I read the entries, I can relive those days. It isn't a mystery why I was happy. My health had bounced back from the toxic new-construction school I attended when I was eleven. It had been a couple of years since Dad stopped beating me, so I was no longer afraid of physical violence from day to day. For much of the year I was fifteen, Dad was blessedly gone, living by himself in Germany and doing research for another book. I lived at home with my siblings and my mother, and I enjoyed school, homework, and hobbies. I loved my job in a sandwich shop, where I finally got enough to eat after years of lean meals at home. Just as happens when poor people enter the military, all that salami, ham, and tuna fish salad corrected undiagnosed and long-term nutritional deficiencies, so I felt fantastic. I started jogging for exercise and to alleviate menstrual pain.

Alongside this basic contentment, my deepest source of happiness and joy was boys. Boys were wonderful, delightful, and fascinating creatures who smelled nice and who I loved to look at and talk to. Unlike girls, they didn't care if my clothes weren't just right or if my family was odd. I liked boys my own age and also young men who were a good bit older. I liked popular boys and also boys who weren't part of the "in" crowd. I repeatedly made boyfriends of my girlfriends' older brothers and Kirsten's male friends. I got crushes on my parents' friends, male teachers, customers at work, neighbors, and people I met wherever I went. When these people looked at me, I could tell that they didn't judge but liked me right back. I went from fun to fun to fun, from my job where there were boys, to school where there were boys, to dates and phone calls with boys. I was over the top boy crazy.

When I was fifteen, Bill was a friend in his early thirties who lived upstairs in the seven-unit apartment building my parents owned. Mrs. Jones was my math teacher. Lynn and Mike were boyfriends who were in college. Ginger and Tiny were my good friends.

I wrote in my journal:

*Jan 1, 1978*
*Yesterday Bill and I went for a 5 mi. hike then I went to Tiny's party. Mason, Bob, and Will were there. Shot fire-crackers and drank a teeny bit of champagne. Tiny drank a lot and giggled and Ginger got bombed, puked for a while, and then passed out on the couch. I smooched with Mason a little and he drove me home at 3:45. He was being very affectionate. The front door was locked and I had to climb*

*in the window in Amy's room. She woke up and I wished
her a happy new year.*

*Got out of bed this morning at 10:30. Bill and I went
for another walk—this time down to the river and back—I
was so tired.*

*At 5:00 I went over to Tiny's and she & Ginger &
I went to see "The World's Greatest Lover," with Gene
Wilder—unbelievable but funny. Got back—went upstairs
and said hello to Bill—and took a bath (desperately needed).*

*I called Mike and asked, "How are you doing?"
whereupon he answered, "What does it matter to you?"
Later in a very brief conversation he said that he wanted
to have a talk with me soon and that it was important. I
said, "OK." He sounded really pissed. Maybe I don't care.
But I think I do.*

*Dad is coming back tonight. Mom is at the airport
right now waiting for him. Things will be very different
around here after he comes back.*

*Jan 2, 1978*
*Dad was home this morning and I hugged him in the
kitchen. He got terribly emotional—started crying even—I
was touched. He had a moustache and showed me a jade
necklace that he bought for Mom. I thought it was ugly.*

*I have a lot of trouble deciding what people at school think
of me. I've decided that I use schoolwork and books as a crutch.
I'm not very social. Mrs. Jones's mother is dying and J. is
upset. I told her about my grandfather and how he died while
coming home to his family on Christmas, and that seemed to
cheer her up a little. We're having X-mas this evening.*

*I seem to spend a lot of time looking at myself. I haven't
run for days even though Bill and I have walked—he has*

*had sinus infections, a sinus headache (for the last two wks.), etc. Must get out.*

*Haven't called Lynn yet—no reason to and nothing to say. Lynn is a little bit too gorgeous.*

Later that month I learned that the reason I had always been terrible at any social or sporting activity that involved catching things out of the air was because I had poor vision in one eye and had no depth perception. When my friend Bill took me to the Registry of Motor Vehicles to get my driving learner's permit, the woman behind the counter cut off the vision to my right eye to test my left eye. All I saw was yellow blobs. "What letters?" I repeatedly said when prompted, as she evidently kept making the black print letters bigger and bigger. "I don't see any letters." I honestly had no idea that my vision was defective, which it had evidently been since birth. Either my eyes had never been tested, or they had and my parents ignored the results.

*Jan 11, 1978*

*Nothing happened in school today except yet more pressure for exams was applied. Loaned Randolph twenty cents.*

*At the bus stop Dorothy F. asked me, "Are you and Mike still dating?" right out of the blue. I could have hit her! I said only, "I've talked with him recently and nothing else." How obnoxious!*

*Bill gave me these little aquamarine earrings for Christmas and birthday. I love them! Yesterday he and I went down to get my permit and we couldn't because I am blind in one eye. It was the craziest scene. Also, folk dancing was canceled. I haven't run since Sunday and Dad's still in LA.*

Lucy was a school friend with a droll sense of humor, who was a member of a girls' social club called Les Coquettes. There were rumors around school that recent pledges to Les Coquettes had been forced to strip down to bra and underpants and lie in the back of a pickup truck. Then, the older girls poured ketchup and flour over them. When Lucy tried to persuade me to become a pledge, I read on her face the desire to see me screaming and writhing while trapped and covered in filth, but I was not able to fully articulate this premonition in my journal.

*Jan 13, 1978*
*Friday at last! Wet walk to school. Then Lucy tried on and off all day to convince me to take a bid from Les Coquettes. No way!! Don't have the money, time, nor the need for support. They can just go to hell.*

*Mailed a letter to Mason today and also my SAT scores. Went up to see Bill after din. but had to leave twenty min. later because I was babysitting for the Vanderwoods. He told me that he wished I would babysit for him once in a while.*

*While babysitting, I spent most of my time feeding boogers to this bored-stiff goldfish in a bowl and eating potato chips. $3.50 for 3½ hours. I'm going to have to raise my rates. Went to see if I could visit Bill afterward at ten fifteen, but his car wasn't there even though his lights were on. Snuck around the building feeling creepy until I got sick of it and went in. Friday the 13th. How about that? And nothing's happened. No word from Mike, and he was supposed to be home today. Maybe he's playing hard to get.*

Around this time Bill and I had sex, the first time for me. We occasionally did it again over the next few months. My parents had no interest in where I was from day to day, so I was not afraid of getting caught. We lounged around in his apartment, and he would sometimes cook us meals. I was motivated by curiosity and a sense of adventure rather than romance or passion. Bill was short-ish and fat-ish, and I was unimpressed by the act itself. Now, forty years later and considering our age difference, I see that although I felt neither coerced nor exploited at the time, there had been earlier signs that he was grooming me for a sexual relationship. Probably this mature man saw what I could not: that I, a beautiful girl, was alone in the world and willing to pay an unfair price for friendship. But that age-old story is not the one that I'm telling here.

*Feb 8, 1978*
*Watched Bill cook fried chicken and wrote a letter to Lynn. Kirsten and I had another bathroom scene. She tells me to hurry, and when it takes me twenty min. to take a bath and wash my hair, she yells at me and calls me an absolute bitch. I didn't even get a chance to brush my teeth.*

*I've thought about it, and decided that it is true that Kirsten has more clothes and more in general. I hate to see myself as the "deprived second child," but sometimes I feel like I am. Mom never buys me any clothes or anything (one example is that her Fabergé and Cologne posters got backed, and that cost $22.00) and I've just gotten to the point where if I want anything, I buy it myself. It is an automatic train of thought. Why does Kirsten get in these moods where she hates me and calls me a bitch, etc.? These bathroom scenes occur regularly and seem to be almost setups. She waits until I am in, tells me in a pained voice to "please hurry up," and then ten min. later starts banging regularly on the door.*

*I'm still sick.*

I worked twenty hours a week in the sandwich shop and was deeply happy at that job. Despite being disappointed in my first experiences of sex, I was still man crazy. Jack was a handsome, flirty, married man in his late thirties who lived down the street.

*May 2, 1978*
*Lynn D. called me at work and wanted to come to town tonight and go out with me but I said no I wanted to run and couldn't stay out till one on a weeknight. I'll see him later. I got home and ran, and Glenn called and I talked with him for a while. I want to see him sometime soon. I went out to Carousel with Randolph last Sat. night and he tried to kiss me, but I wouldn't let him and turned my cheek to him. He was embarrassed, and I think he likes me. He's a nice guy but I'm not in love with him. Glenn was nice to talk to. Haven't talked to Marty but I still like him because I think of him all the time.*

*I came home and skateboarded for a while, I'm getting better, then did a wash, took a bath and washed my hair, and went to bed. Altogether a very productive day. I'm leading a good life.*

*I like Joe, but he doesn't pay much attention to me.*
*I also like Jack.*

*I was just looking over my entry and thinking that I must be a very male-oriented person because I can't seem to find very much to say about very many female friends. That's funny. I have crushes on all these men.*

These were the years I was creating the person I should have been for the rest of my life. When I was fourteen and fifteen, I was healthy and was safe at home. I had enough to eat and a quiet place to sleep, and I felt love within my family. I was busy during the day with hobbies, school, and a job, and I excelled at these activities. I have all of these things, or reasonable replacements for them, in my current middle-aged life. But when I was fourteen and fifteen, there was also a magic ingredient, which was the company of boys.

Now that I am fifty-five, what is the special sauce, meaning the age-appropriate replacement for the magic of boys? It could be clarity of thought and the full acceptance of my losses, blah, blah, blah. But where is the joy going to come from? The past forty years have turned me from a sweet natured and generous child to a skeptical and inward looking woman. For the next little while and until I am fully satisfied, the special sauce will include all the brutal and nihilistic revenge that it is possible for me to either imagine or inflict without going to jail. From social butterfly at fifteen to vindictive crone at fifty-five—those are surely platonic ideals, so maybe my life will finally make some sense. I will mine the dullness and struggles of the lost forty years for messages I previously ignored and memories of unkindness that still rankle, and from these lessons and memories I will craft truth, then resolution, and, finally, righteous justice.

# Chapter 11 - Brain Stimulation

∽

When I was fourteen or fifteen, apropos of nothing and without any agenda, I asked my mother about my collapse as an infant. She told me I had mysteriously become comatose and that I had been in the hospital for several weeks. The cause was unknown, and she and Dad thought I would die. When I came home from the hospital, it was a long time before I acted normal again. Then, lightly, she said, "Well, anyway, your father and I always thought it stimulated your brain." She spoke the words without effort of recall, and I intuited that their conversations about the aftereffects had been distant and also recent. She looked down as people do when they are hiding something, and bizarrely, she giggled.

While observing as best I can the effects of chemical exposures on my abilities and activities, I have noticed that the dulling impairment of a period of exposure is followed by a resurgence of creativity and enthusiasm. Parts of my brain are stimulated into extra neurological activity as they recover from damage. This is what my parents saw as I was growing up. It wasn't that the one-time damage and impairment from the initial injury resulted in a permanent change to intelligence and creativity. She was telling me that the reinjuries they observed were followed by periods of unusual mental exuberance. Why else would it have been a recurrent topic of conversation? If there had only been the one initial injury and recovery, they would not have needed to discuss it repeatedly. As Mom looked down and away and giggled, she retreated into secret reflection. She seemed uncomfortable, so I didn't press her further.

After I became so ill at age forty-eight and having read articles that conjectured that certain Iraq War veterans developed sensitivities from chemical exposures, I began to suspect my illness during infancy was the underlying cause for my new broad-based chemical intolerance. I cast my mind over long-ago conversations with members of my family. Earlier, I had assumed that my parents hadn't made the connection between the first event, my chronic health problems, and then, later, my complete disability. But this conversation with my mother haunted me. As I repeatedly replayed it, I connected thoroughly with the information I intuited all those years ago but had had no context for. I allowed for a possibility that now seems obvious; namely, Mom and Dad had a secret regarding my early illness, they jointly observed the long-term effects on my health, and they hid these observations from me. Nothing else makes sense. As I write these words, this conclusion makes complete sense.

How do you tell a child she has a physical weakness that is not readily apparent, recurs at intervals, results in cognitive and behavioral impairments, and is the cause for other symptoms, like bad sleep, lack of physical stamina, terrible menstrual pain, and noise sensitivity? What if common sense indicates that of course the chemical exposure had weakened the child, but contemporaneous medical science has no name for the effect and denies the connection between chemical exposures and subsequent chemical intolerance? What if it was your husband's fault, and, if you finally admit the damage to the child, she will eventually figure out it happened through his carelessness? What if on top of all this, you have not loved this child since you thought she would die as an infant?

Dad came home from Germany partway through that school year and took up creepy habits. He was a beautiful man with a large and well-formed penis, and he would "accidentally" show me his penis by leaving the bath with a loosely draped towel that then fell off. Or, he walked through the apartment naked but cupping his genitals in one hand for only part of the time, or he excessively fiddled with his penis or balls near me while wearing running shorts. I don't think he was trying to groom me for real sex. Instead, he was enjoying the low and nasty "shock and awe" effect, flasher-on-the-street style. I remember him looking closely into my face when he did these things, while I tried to look away. Possibly for him this was a new not-nice way to connect with me, since he had stopped beating me a few years earlier. I didn't see his penis as often as I did my mother's breasts, but I could pick it out of a lineup, no problem. I ignored these episodes and considered them just another manifestation of his general unpleasantness and weirdness.

I was accepted into a six-week summer academic program called Governor's School, which ran at a college in a beautiful coastal city. High school students of exceptional achievement from throughout the state were invited to live in the dorms and take special classes for free. We had a lot of time to explore the city and also pursue the nontraditional assignments. I was still boy crazy. My journal entries are filled with movies, plays, outings, discussions, and smooches, with many different young men.

I started hanging out with a college-age brother of a high school friend, and then I spent one night at his apartment off campus. The next morning there were city police knocking at his door looking for me. I didn't have any idea what the fuss was about, but evidently when I went missing there had been a lot of fuss. I went to see the head of the school and apologized to this man for not letting anyone know where I was. I refused to tell him whether or not I had had sex, and he seemed genuinely confused by my attitude that it wasn't anyone else's business where I went or what I did. On my part, I was flabbergasted to learn that there was oversight of the children and that there existed an authority figure who had an interest in my movements. He kept me in his office chatting for a while, which must have been to make sure I was OK and had not been coerced. There was less than a week left to the program, so despite the trouble I had caused, I was not kicked out.

My life changed hugely when I got home from Governor's School. That day, about a month before my sixteenth birthday, my father told me I had to move out of the family home. He said my presence was deeply upsetting to my mother and that she felt I was deliberately coming between them. Also, he said that I was a disruptive force in their marriage and in the household, and they needed me to leave. I was to move into an empty apartment upstairs with my older sister, who was taking a year off before college, and I was not to approach my mother or speak to her. Dad refused to give examples of what I had said or done and instead implied that I already knew. I was thunderstruck and had no idea what he was talking about. I associated their decision with my night missing, but that episode was not mentioned. In fact, my parents had never told us that sex was sinful or deserving of punishment. Now I see that Mom had either noticed or intuited Dad's feelings about me and had twisted her own feelings of loss and sexual frustration into a belief that I wanted to steal Dad's sexual attentions away from her. Given how deeply oblivious I was back then to the strongest and most hidden currents in our home, there is a good chance that Dad's behavior had been going on for years in more subtle ways and that her resentment toward me had been building for quite a while.

Now I also see that my sexuality was a secondary issue. My mother had never recovered from my early illness. She wasn't able to love me again after the twin shocks of thinking I was going to die and then thinking I was permanently mentally impaired. As she observed recurring signs of the damage she and Dad had inadvertently caused, she was tormented and hated me for the way I made her feel. When she looked at me, she saw a selfish, hurtful troublemaker whom she was justified in treating badly.

Although I was a show-off and full of myself, I wasn't careless or cruel. I did not do drugs or alcohol. I made good grades while working twenty hours a week, and I blew the top off of standardized tests. I made bead jewelry, sewed clothing, and had a passion for propagating houseplants. I jogged regularly, did more than my share of housework, and kept a tidy room. I also had no interest in the inner workings of their marriage and in no way did I ever flirt with Dad. When she looked at me and saw a monster, she was delusional.

Mom and Dad found my frenetic social life disconcerting and distracting. Neither of them wanted the responsibility for controlling or limiting my behavior, but it bothered them that I was so active and having so much fun. Dad liked to be the center of attention and had fundamental distress when someone near him was focused on other activities and other people, so my social life was especially painful for him.

The arrangement in which my older sister and I lived in a separate apartment suited my parents in practical ways. For the two years since Dad bought the building and we moved into it, my parents had struggled with space limitations. For a while,

Hunter's bed was in a strange airless cubbyhole off a center hall, and, when Dad was in Germany, Mom slept in a bed in a corner of the living room. If we two older girls moved out, then Hunter and Amy could have their own rooms and Mom and Dad could have their own bedroom and regain conjugal privacy. It had already been decided that Kirsten, then almost eighteen, would take a year off before starting college. Mom had gotten her a job working in a friend's law office. Kirsten could have lifestyle independence to match her new quasi-professional job, and, if I lived with her, she would be safer in the apartment.

Dad felt low when he was alone too much and had become depressed while living by himself in Germany. He knew he needed Mom and his marriage not to be miserable. He also knew he had behaved in sexually inappropriate ways toward me and that it would be better for him if he and I were not living in the same place. After a year away, he wasn't secure about his status and was desperate to be welcomed back into my mother's gracious and comforting sphere. Mom's price for renewed intimacy and affection was that Dad agree I was a malevolent force within their marriage. Years before, when I was ill as an infant, she was forced to choose between me and her marriage, and she chose her marriage. Now she compelled Dad to make a similar choice. She also told him he had to convey their shared belief that my destructive impact was deliberate and a reflection of my bad character. He agreed to her demand that I leave their home, and, when I asked why, he followed the script they had agreed to. As a result of his loyalty, Mom and Dad felt a renewed closeness and commitment to each other after their year apart.

Neither of my parents was willing to see a family therapist because of laziness and also because of guilt over their mistreatment of their children. Dad didn't want to spend the money and also didn't want anyone telling him what to do, and Mom feared social shame and lacked confidence in her own profession. They were unwilling to do the heavy lifting to build a healthier family in the future and were unable to manage my departure in a way that wasn't hurtful to me. It was as if they had taken all of their own mistakes and conjugal disappointments, bundled and molded them into the shape of a monkey backpack, strapped it to my back, spit and kicked at me and the monkey for a little while, and then tried to set us both on fire. It wasn't fair or nice, but it worked for them.

I felt confusion and shame after my parents kicked me out of the house, and I doubted my own character and intentions. I wish that back then someone had shared with me the certain truth that a high proportion of people are neurotic, lack kindness, or both. When I was young, I read so much romantic literature that I believed the world was good and that people were motivated by the desire to be just. Now I know that most people are selfish and do not hesitate to be unkind. Both because we humans are tender lumps of meat in a chemical soup and also because we are social creatures susceptible to either accidental or deliberate damage from others, we should stay home more, where we are relatively safe.

If you just stay home, you can live a prairie lifestyle in which interactions with others are infrequent and therefore cherished. You will have more time for useful reflection and can make better choices regarding whom you want to be with. On those rare occasions when you meet someone of quality, you will have more time and space to appreciate them. Possibly there are members of your family you should offload. Try to see these people clearly and get rid of them.

Lay off the romantic literature and movies, and look at the world with clarity. It is a chemical world, not a world where human constructs of virtue are rewarded. It is a world where the consumer goods that you bring into your home contain neuro-disruptors and hormone disruptors that are insufficiently regulated and tested, a world where the selfishness and stupidity of major corporations mean that we all are bathed in masking fragrances that are making us and our loved ones ill. Get rid of excess people and excess stuff in the interest of your well-being, and acknowledge that the chemical realities of your environment are ultimately the most important realities. The shade of your lipstick and the style of your car are nothing compared to whether or not you get a good night's sleep or whether or not your child has asthma.

# Chapter 12 - Senior Year

Kirsten and I lived together in a mostly empty three-bedroom apartment that next year. We didn't pay rent, but we did pay our own telephone and electric bills and we bought and prepared our own food, separately. Lunch at my public high school's cafeteria cost fifty-five cents and extra milk four cents, so even though the cafeteria was social suicide for a middle-class white person, I ate lunch there by myself most school days. I also got free meals at my job at the sandwich shop. In addition to working at the sandwich shop, I worked as a janitor for Dad in the apartment building. I saved money for college.

When Kirsten and I lived together, we led separate lives. I had a new college-age boyfriend and friends at work, while Mom often took Kirsten to lunch or clothes shopping for her job at the law office. Mom didn't visit in the apartment, but the two of them spent a lot of time together. I didn't often see my younger siblings. In my journal, I complain about Dad being unpleasant, about Amy stealing my socks from the basement laundry area, and about Kirsten borrowing my clothes without asking and then damaging them.

I still loved my mother and wanted to be with her. Because I did not understand what I could have done to cause her discomfort or threaten her marriage, I suppressed the evidence of her dislike. Instead, I attributed the distance between us to mysterious and unknowable family dynamics. I believed she still loved me and that, for some adult reason that I was incapable of understanding, we needed to be apart. Now I see that this distance was a profound relief for her. She had made herself believe what she told Dad about my intentions and personality. She and Kirsten became even closer, their bond strengthened by Kirsten's misery at still being single while I had an excess of boyfriends. When circumstances did bring Mom and me together, she was civil but distant. I told her I needed to get fitted for a diaphragm, and she gritted it out and brought me to a doctor for this purpose.

By myself, I gathered and completed college applications for Harvard, Duke, Yale, and Rice, carefully filling out the forms and completing the essays. I paid the application fees myself, each one representing many hours of my minimum-wage job. Despite the inferiority of my education in the public schools of that time and place, I was accepted at all four colleges. Two of them offered partial tuition support based on my academic achievements in high school. I decided to go to Harvard. Kirsten planned to attend Georgetown University.

Toward the end of that school year, after I stole one of Kirsten's good friends and turned him into my boyfriend, I complained in my journal that she was resentful and did a pulse check on my own moral development:

> *Kirsten has been feeling (and acting) very hostile toward me lately. I think she sees herself as the victim in our relationship with the family. She thinks that she has been made*

to feel inferior (Harvard vs. Georgetown) and also generally mistreated by Dad. I haven't talked to her for at least a week. Dad on the other hand is all ready to assume the martyr position again. Everyone treats me like the bad guy, it's clear you all want me to leave, etc. Making anything that is said to him, especially by me, for reasons I have yet to pinpoint, subject to an exact scrutinization for him to determine if it was a remark undermining him in any way.

My main concern right now is what kind of person I am, how nice I am to people. My family (except Hunter) makes me feel obnoxious and unpleasant (I am willing to accept that possibility). Amy irritates, the notable things Dad says to me concern my being difficult and threatening in the household, Kirsten is moody and resentful. Mom is merely insensitive at times when I need a kind word or gesture. Maybe the whole family has come to regard me the same way I realize I regard Amy. I treat her as someone who has a lot of support within herself and doesn't really need it from me. (She's eleven.) She knows that she's beautiful, intelligent (even brilliant perhaps), well-read, so I don't tell her that because I'm afraid she will want to flaunt it more than she already does. What she needs, I think, as I do, is guidance and encouragement on the moral side, the human-relations side. Actually, I don't steal things. But I do have serious doubts about my relationships with other people. The conclusion to all this, which occurred to me back on the previous page, is that I need to leave my family and build relationships with other people so I can judge for myself how I do in that respect. I need to be removed from previous prejudices that the family might have against me and try to prove to myself that I'm good or at least that my attempts at success along that road have resulted in positive change.

I'm proud of myself for taking charge of the direction of my education and paying my own expenses that year. But my journal entries are filled with self-doubt and don't have the joy of the previous year. I didn't know it at the time, but I had lost my mother for good, and this loss caused a shadow of sadness and emptiness that has followed me to this day.

# Chapter 13 - High School Clothes

Our high school clothes can tell our story for us. I dreamt of long-lasting and modest clothing that expressed quiet homage to my body without celebrating sexuality. In photo after photo, including each of my four yearbook photos, I'm wearing scavenged items from Kirsten's friends via Kirsten's reject pile. I remember clearly each item shown in these photographs, as my wardrobe was tiny. With limited success, I repurposed some of my father's worn dress shirts by shortening the body and sleeves, cutting off the collar, and then tying them at my waist. In one junior year grip-n-grin, as the governor of the state shakes my hand and hands me a piece of paper in recognition of some sort of academic achievement, I'm wearing a gathered off-white dress that I bought for the occasion. I took a city bus by myself to a local department store to find it. I didn't like the dress much, but it was the best I could manage with my babysitting earnings and one of a few clothing articles I as a child ever possessed that was purchased retail, full price, for me as the original owner.

I knew I was not conforming to social norms but did not shave my legs or other parts of my body because shaving seemed like gratuitous mutilation. Even in my early teens, I intuited that the power that came from high heels and revealing clothing was a false, destructive, and superficial power. Being too pretty attracted the wrong kind of attention both inside the house and outside of it, from women and from men. I sensed that if I were to crank up my sex appeal through the beauty routines that were standard for my friends and classmates, my family wouldn't protect me and I would be vulnerable to predation that would in a way be my own fault. I wore a tiny bit of lip color or mascara only sometimes and did not use any styling products or styling tools on my hair.

I attended a handful of the formal dances that were a main-stay of the white upper-class social scene at that time, and I have couple's photographs of me and each of my dates from each party. These photos show me in one of Mom's work dresses, then in a dress that belonged to one of Kirsten's friends, and then in a borrowed light blue silk Chinese embroidered jacket with shiny cream-colored pants. I looked fine. This last outfit, which I liked a lot, made my date for that dance express repeated and vigorous bitterness, both during the evening and afterward, because he had expected me to wear a dress.

During the last months of my junior year, as the prom approached, I had a huge crush on a senior boy who was way out of my league. But, I could tell he liked me at least a little bit. In a gesture that was boldly gender-bending for that time and place, I bought two tickets to the prom and asked him to go with me. I ended up asking him a few times because of his apparent ambivalence; then, he finally turned me down in a definitive manner. Disgusted by his rejection of me, burdened by two expensive and wasted tickets, and then inspired by a cast-off blouse with vertical ruffles that was in Mom's closet, I walked to the local formal wear shop and rented a pair of men's tuxedo trousers, a bow-tie, and some shiny black shoes. I went to the prom with a girlfriend in a paroxysm of further gender-bending exuberance. I remember worrying about being asked to leave the prom because of my outfit and at the same time feeling adventurous and defiant. This was the Deep South in 1978, and I was fifteen years old.

A year and a half after the governor shook my hand, photos show me again wearing the off-white gathered dress, this time at my high school graduation. I am cheerfully standing tall, slender arms at my sides, the dress tied with a same-fabric belt around my narrow waist. The sleeves come halfway down my upper arms, and the dress falls to my mid calf. I look just fine.

# Chapter 14 - Left College

I don't remember Dad being mean to Mom when we were kids, but we still felt sorry for her for having to live with him. Dad put pressure on her to keep household expenses to a minimum, so it seemed to be his choice, not hers, that we weren't well-fed and had bad clothes. I imagined she wanted us to look nice and be properly nourished but was unwilling to defy him and risk family strife. Just as it was hard for me to make and keep friends because he was ill-tempered and unreasonable, she also had shame and difficulty making good friends. We children understood her to be under continual stress and pressure in her life with him. We thought she was a saint for sacrificing her own happiness to keep the family together and provide us with a home. Probably everyone who knew the two of them socially, as well as members of their own birth families, saw their marriage in this same light.

Much, much later, when they separated en route to divorce after fifty years of marriage, Mom left their house permanently after an unpleasant scene in which Dad shouted at her, among other bitter recriminations, "You ruined my life!" We children laughed at him behind his back for thinking anyone would believe this for a second. Now I'm not so inclined to see her purely as an innocent and him purely as a beast. Maybe what my father meant in his inchoate rage that last time they were alone together was that his damage, both inherent to himself and also inflicted on others, served her purposes: that she was able to craft the whole and virtuous person she wanted to be because he was a foil, and that his generalized crazy behavior was a smokescreen for her own cowardice and empty core.

When I was in high school and college, we children knew Mom went to see a therapist on a regular basis and that his name was Bruce. We thought he was a friendly acquaintance of the family, even though we had never met him, and that Mom derived well-deserved comfort and companionship from her chats with him. We knew this long-term friendship was expensive, but we believed since she earned her own money, she could spend it on whatever she wanted.

The apartment building threw off a lot of cash income. When I was in my early teens, Dad transferred one-fifth of the ownership to each of his four children so that rental income would be taxed at their lower rates, leaving him more cash to pay for their future educations. The building was held in a family limited partnership with each child's interest kept in trust until he or she turned twenty-one. Dad explained to us that at that point, each share would no longer be controlled by the trustee, who happened to be Mom, and would instead be ours for our own disposition. When I went to Harvard as a freshman in the fall of 1979 right after I turned seventeen, he sent Harvard the required amounts for tuition, room, and board. He also paid for occasional items, like airfare home for Christmas. Despite his lofty intentions to secure his children's financial futures by setting up the tax-minimizing scheme, he continued to be ungracious when it came to smaller practical matters, like schoolbooks, supplies, winter clothing, or incidentals. I got a job washing dishes in the freshman dining hall and, later, another cleaning offices on campus.

During my freshman year at Harvard, all indications were that my time there would be a modest success. I made good grades, had friends, and had lots of boyfriends. I fancied myself an entrepreneur and adventuress when, a few times that year and by myself, I took the train to New York City, stayed in the YMCA downtown, shopped for beads in the wholesale button district, and explored the great city. I was making the best of my circumstances, but my journal entries are depressing to read now. I frequently wrote about confusion, especially concerning my parents and my own self-worth. The person who wrote these entries was completely different from the girl two years before who had written about all the boys she liked and all the fun she was having.

When I started college, I telephoned my mother once a week because that seemed like the right thing to do. I called her collect, meaning that the charges went to their phone bill, not mine. At age seventeen with a minimum wage job washing dishes, it didn't occur to me that I might pay for them. This went on for several weeks, until Dad telephoned me and told me to stop calling Mom collect. His tone was abrupt, as if he were talking to a neighbor whom he just discovered had been dumping dog shit in his bushes. I wasn't sure at the time if his emphasis was that he didn't want to pay for the calls or that Mom didn't want to talk to me, and I felt confused. Now I think it was both. Afterward I spoke to them on the phone only infrequently.

Another time I wrote my grandmother on my mother's side a longish letter because I fancied she was my friend and took an interest in my thoughts and activities. My mother called me a couple of weeks later and told me she didn't think such long letters to Grandma were a good idea and that shorter letters were better. She conveyed that I had imposed on Grandma and shown a lack of consideration. I felt wounded and confused and wasn't sure what the real message was. I still feel the shock and hurt of both of these conversations. Now I see that they were operating with a secret agenda to diminish my presence in their lives and that these ongoing and meaningful contacts I was trying to establish as I moved away from home were exactly what they didn't want.

In the fall of 1980, when I was eighteen and a college sophomore, I became ill with the first major chemical reinjury of my adult life. As happened when I was eleven and became ill from the German school, and also later in different job environments, the symptoms were neurological and developed gradually. I had terribly disrupted sleep, extreme sensitivity to noise, and non-stop anxiety. Because I believed that to be unhappy was to be a failure, I was self-conscious around my friends, dorm mates, and classmates. My skin and surface muscles ached, and I felt I was moving through mists of discomfort and pain. In addition to jogging several miles a few times a week, I started swimming a mile every day so that simple exhaustion would force me to sleep better. This extreme exercise routine didn't help. One night there was a strange episode after my roommate woke me up repeatedly in an inconsiderate fashion. She kept climbing in and out of our bunk bed as she forgot this or that while she prepared for sleep. Apparently, I cursed violently in frustration for a while, not at her but into the dark room. My response was not reasonable, and I had no memory of it afterward, ever. This event damaged our friendship and made me secretly wonder about my own mental balance.

I talked to my father a few times about how miserable I was but was only able to define the condition in terms of unhappiness, social anxiety, and the strong feeling that what was special about college was being wasted since I was unable to enjoy it. I did not identify the symptoms as neurological, and neither did anyone else. I felt unable to continue living in the dorm and unable to continue being at college. Dad suggested that I go on a few long walks to consider the best decision, which I did without gaining any insight, and then, in a later conversation, he said I could move back to their home. I finished that term and left school before the start of the second semester. Remembering the continual movement in the dorm of workmen with paint buckets and other construction supplies, I now know that chemicals from renovation in and around my suite, possibly compounded by the heavily chlorinated swimming pool where I swam almost daily, had made me ill. At the time, the cause was considered to be psychological, meaning personality weakness and lack of resilience of an unspecified nature.

As I moved home, my mother moved into an empty house about a mile away that Dad had bought as an investment rental property. There was no explanation for her departure. I didn't see her often, but I do remember one visit to her in that house, during which she seemed agitated and uncomfortable with my company. The chitchat was strained. She interpreted my observations and commentary in ways I didn't intend, which then caused offense. I felt affection toward her and accepted this odd behavior as I had always accommodated her apparent distance and evasion around me. Shortly after I moved home, Dad started to put pressure on me to leave. I was eighteen years old. On my own, I found a couple of jobs and an apartment, and, as I moved out, Mom moved back in. Neither of them gave me any money, furniture, or other assistance for these changes in my life.

Once during this time, I needed to see a dentist and had no way to get there. Dad drove me across town complaining all the way about having to do it. By the time the dentist was done with me, Dad had worked himself into a frenzy of resentment and frustration. As we drove back and he went on about how he had better things to do than this, foam pockets formed in the corners of his mouth and spittle droplets sprayed on the steering wheel. Then, during a paroxysm of agitation, he accelerated into the car in front of him, smashing the back of its trunk. It was hysterically funny and totally his fault.

# Chapter 15 - Bruce

Mom arranged for me to talk to her therapist, Bruce. This visit with Bruce was a source of wonderment then and later. I had always thought of Bruce as an auspicious and friendly persona, someone who was able to lift the burdens of my mother's life a little, and someone from whom she got gentle encouragement and support. I looked forward to basking in his cheerful and encouraging presence myself. I had been disappointed with my college experience and was working hard on putting together a life for myself as a (temporary, I hoped) college dropout.

My mother waited in the reception area while I met with Bruce. He was younger than Mom, bearded, and a little pudgy, and looked much as I thought he would. I came prepared to talk about my time at college, the nature of my friendships and boyfriends, and my hopes for the future, but Bruce had no interest in these subjects. When I tried to discuss what I thought was important about myself, Bruce kept turning the conversation back to Mom and Dad.

I didn't pay attention or devote to memory his exact questions because I was mystified by their overall intent. I remember him asking about what I had thought of my parents when I was a young child. Also, what did I now think the two of them were like when they were alone together? Then, there were variations on these themes as he asked me to describe their relationship and tried to assess how much I knew about obscure aspects of their relationship with me and of our history together. I think now that I forgot most of what he said because of my deep confusion about his intentions. A little ways in, I realized he was pumping me for information on behalf of Mom. When I discerned that the conversation had not been arranged to benefit me personally, I was disappointed but trusted that the questions were intended to help her. I answered them as best I could.

With me, he was not the friendly and supportive person I had expected but was instead cagey, with body language that indicated he was uncomfortable. I remember him crossing his arms and looking around his office and out the window as he searched for variations to the questions he had already asked. He didn't seem to like me or be on my side, and yet I had never met the man before. I wondered at his apparent antipathy since I knew I was not a selfish or destructive person and instead wished my mother well and loved her deeply. At the end of the session with Bruce, I ended up feeling worked over, isolated, and disappointed not to have received any connection or comfort.

For decades I didn't trust my own intuition, by which I mean my ability to read and interpret the fine muscles in someone else's face, their eye movements, or subtle tones and pacing in their voice, along with shifts in body chemistry as they exude almost undetectable aromatic indicators of their true emotions. Sadly, I'm sure I still lack the capacity to take these messages in, and I certainly can't claim the ability to overcome my own prejudices and desires enough to translate these messages into useful information. But I would be a stupid person indeed if my past suffering didn't help me see people and the world more clearly now than I did then. At the time, I sensed between Mom and Bruce a shared understanding about a tricky and devious endeavor with results I would not be privy to. Now, many years later, I know what they were trying to achieve.

My visit with Bruce is one of the keys to my mother's inner life. She had paid Bruce a lot of money, and, in return, it was Bruce's job to understand her and be on her side. I now believe that she knew I had had an episode of neurological disruption, which she recognized as a recurring manifestation of my childhood chemical injury. She had instructed Bruce to find out what I knew or was likely to figure out about the underlying cause for my condition, which is why he asked so many questions about my childhood memories and impressions of my parents.

She knew she had failed as a human being when she threw me away because she thought I was a dying baby or, later, a disabled baby. She knew when I grew into a beautiful child and later a young woman that the person she invented when she looked at me was a false one. Her redemption from what she saw as her own despicable weakness came from the self-creation of her persona as a kindly and generous wife, mother, and psychotherapist. She wanted Bruce to find out if I was likely to blow her cover.

Was it a breach of professional ethics for Bruce to exploit a vulnerable child as he did? Possibly Mom told him I was sexually promiscuous or that I was a malignant force whose presence weakened her marriage. These were the apparent reasons I had been asked to leave the family home when I was fifteen. Whatever the earlier discussions between Mom and Bruce and however she justified their plans to him, it was clear the two of them had a secret and shared motivation that involved Mom's self-interest, not my mental health. He was so uncomfortable because partway through our meeting he realized he was sitting in front of a well-meaning child who had been ill and that he was doing a dirty job and getting shit on his shoes.

∞

A mother's love for a child is a great gift, one I never had. It changes the child from a lonely creature in a hostile world to a lucky being in a world that is basically safe. How do I, after being alone and unlucky, somehow recreate myself as someone who is, if not smiled upon by the world, at least not kicked in the teeth? What are the touchstones of truth, understanding, or wisdom that can help me build a new life?

The only chance I have of recasting myself as a lucky person is if I stay home. It is dangerous for me outside of the house, with auto fumes, laundry vents, bank lobby carpets, cleaning supplies, and people who smell of fragranced products. Even at home, there are dangers including books, consumer goods, hobby supplies, alcoholic beverages, personal care products, magazines—all the fun stuff. They all contain substances that destroy my nervous system and therefore my true self. If I am to build a new life in which I force myself to be lucky in contradiction to a lifetime of bad fortune, I can't rely on the usual distractions and consolations.

Other people have achieved contentment and even accomplishment from staying home. Nelson Mandela, Marcel Proust, Emily Dickinson—these superior and enlightened people were able to realize their true natures even as they were confined. Perhaps confinement forced them to rise above the concerns of the average human. Whatever my initial gifts, my neurology is now too damaged for me to achieve greatness. However, quiet contentment and a gradual increase in wellness are yet within my scope.

When Husband and I were forced to move out of the Boston area by smells in the neighborhood and in our home, we bought an unusually large old house in a small town. After this house came on the market and we went out to take a look at it, I wrote to a friend who was familiar with the town and the house that Husband and I had decided against taking the bus to crazy-town, meaning we had decided not to take the house. But then circumstances changed our minds, and we bought it as a fuck-you gesture against how small our lives had become. We know it isn't ours, but only ours to take care of for a while.

Our house was built by a seed-and-feed magnate of the late nineteenth century. Like other commercial barons of the time, he wanted an enormous and beautiful testament to his own success as well as reassurance to current and potential creditors. He had the house overconstructed to the same standard as his grain warehouses, which were scattered around the county next to railroad tracks. High ceilings, sycamore paneled rooms, timber framing so substantial it doesn't make sense, and about a hundred windows, no lie. Husband and I joked that when the magnate ordered up the house, he told his engineers to mow the arboretum. Arts and Crafts bungalow meets the *Titanic*. At considerable trouble and expense, we renovated the house using only nontoxic building materials, and it is a safe place for me to live. We are prepared to spend a disproportionate percentage of our budget on the necessary upkeep, compared to a different housing approach, and we each have a great deal of space for ourselves.

Our other important lifestyle choice is that we eat food of the highest quality, meaning organic, local, and carefully selected ingredients. The "holy shit!" house and the simple yet expensive food are our two luxuries. In cold weather, the thermostat is set to the high fifties during the day and the mid forties at night. We don't have a car. We don't travel or buy new clothes.

I am waiting for my tired spirit to regain enthusiasm for gardening and keeping chickens, and I will then get three to five large-breed hens. My hens will have impossibly strong legs and feet, like rocket thrusters. When I see my gorgeous pets running, their grace and power will make me smile from deep joy, just like the long-dead seed magnate used to smile when he contemplated the massive timbers tucked behind his acres of sycamore paneling.

I am waiting for my tired spirit to regain an interest in learning, and I will pursue internet learning for pleasure. I will study vocabulary, history, science, and the writings of people like Noam Chomsky and Naomi Klein. Among fruiting bushes next to my three-story ship and with a heavy and gentle bird on my lap, after lunch prepared by my cheerful husband and listening to the wisdom of Noam or Naomi on the radio, I will know I have made my own luck.

# Chapter 16 - Visit to Doctor

∽

Recently I went to see my doctor for an annual physical checkup. The waiting room smelled of carpets and fragranced cleaning products, so while I waited I held my half-face respirator up to my face. I was a little low when I first arrived because of my effing period, which blight seemingly refuses to permanently leave my life, and later also because of smells from the waiting room coming through the mask. The doctor's assistant is my age and normally a chatty and cheerful person. Because I was low, I didn't possess the extra attenuation that usually makes me take off the mask fully for a moment to smile at her. Each visit she takes my weight on the way to the examination room, and she must have gathered I wasn't at a hundred percent when I got on the scale without bothering to either put down my bag or take off my coat. Key indicator that a woman has other stuff on her mind: she weighs herself while wearing a winter coat and holding a large handbag. Nurses and aides that we passed in the hallway looked down and away. I knew this wasn't because of my personality and was instead because of the mask, but I still found their evasive looks dismaying. Usually, the assistant calls me "my dear" and "honey," which I find lovely, and tells me about her sex life and female complaints. This time, because I wasn't able to give her a full-face connection, she was more distant.

During our brief interview before the doctor came in, I became more miserable as I realized she was uncomfortable. This feeling of social isolation, plus the poisoning effect of the odors from the waiting room, plus anxiety about the doctor treating my concerns with respect, plus slight shame at the memory of crying the last time I was in his office, all combined to make me truly miserable. I was supposed to be visiting a healer, and instead the experience was depressing me before it had even begun.

The physical exam was unremarkable. The doctor was pleasant and respectful, and I tried not to be weird or demanding. I like this doctor, and he believes my story because he lives in Franklin County and has internalized its humanistic and supportive culture. But the experience was a reminder of how isolating my condition is. I am a social and affectionate creature, so this is hard on me.

Even though I had Husband nearby when I was so ill at forty-eight years old, I felt more alone than I ever had before. Great swaths of the fabric of my life fell away, and I lost connection with memory, hopes for the future, likes and dislikes, a daily routine, friends and colleagues, and interest in the wider world. My mind was a pain-wracked shadow of my normal self. I knew anguish was written all over my face and that other people were made uncomfortable when they looked at me. I was desperate to receive the comfort of basic kindness, but, because I was so deeply impaired, I was unable to generate kindness within others. To be human is to connect with others, and it has seemed to me since that dark time that of all the illnesses, mental impairment must be the most isolating and therefore the most dehumanizing.

The deterioration of the mind is a partial death. Just as someone moving toward full death should be treated with gentleness and kindness, people experiencing the partial death of mental illness or neurological impairment should be treated with excessive gentleness and kindness to console them for their loss of humanity as well as their basic anguish. This is not easy because these people often act badly. Witness my father, who, when he was behaving his worst, jabbered nonsensically (I thought then) about his need for kindness.

These pervasive chemicals in our world are causing people a great deal of undiagnosed mental impairment. The daily news is filled with people acting badly: sending dick pics, shooting strangers, punching people on the street, leaving babies in hot cars, trolling abusively online, hitting people because a fast food order is delayed. These people are impaired because of the fragrance in their laundry detergent, the carpets in their cars, or the additives in their flavored coffee. Just as the chemicals around me made me miserable and addled, the chemicals around these people are making them miserable and addled. This is a completely true and important fact, but the world isn't ready to admit it just yet.

# Chapter 17 - Dad and Money

After I left college midway through my sophomore year and moved back to my hometown ("Hometown," from here on out), I continued to struggle with the long-term health effects of my exposure to toxic building materials in the dorm the previous semester. I had bad sleep, fatigue, and anxiety, which have always been the primary symptoms of a chemical reinjury for me. I built a new life around dance classes, waitressing, teaching aerobic dancing, distance lap swimming, and new friends, mostly male. I was in recovery mode, nursing my wounds from what had been a brutalizing time at school. Even though my apartment was two blocks from my family home, I didn't see my family much. I did not receive guidance or advice from either of my parents.

During my late teens and early twenties, I tried to turn my maternal grandmother into a friend by writing her many times a year. Much later when she was downsizing her home, she returned a packet of these letters, and after she died I got another pile of them. Rereading them now, thirty-five years later, I am struck by how determined and hardworking I am and how forgiving of my parents.

I avoided Dad mostly because that seemed the best approach. The only time in my life I lost my cool with him was after he offered to lend me a copper omelet pan that had always been part of our family kitchen but that he and Mom weren't using at the time. I accepted, but when I came over to get the pan a couple of days later, Dad accused me of stealing it and stealing from their home generally. I lost it and started screaming at him as I left his house. As I walked away from him down the street, I kept crying and screaming at him as he followed me, quiet and looking worried. This episode was important because years later in a legal deposition he testified that I had a history of physical violence. He said that in the past I had been violent toward myself and others. I suppose the closest I had ever gotten was this omelet pan incident, where he provoked me into a verbal rage. Perhaps as time passed, the actuality of my walking away from him and crying transformed in his memory into an event where I was walking toward him and making threatening gestures of some kind. In previous years, he had often accused me of unkindness or bad intentions, when in retrospect it is clear these impulses were what he was feeling. Perhaps during the omelet pan episode he attributed to me violent urges because he felt full of violence himself. Or, maybe in the deposition he lied because he could and that particular lie suited his purpose.

If my parents had been awful all of the time, it would have been easier to leave them behind. However, sometimes they were reasonable and civil, and there were even times when they seemed connected to me as their daughter. I chose to see the sporadic episodes of apparent connectedness and normality as the expression of their true selves, and I downplayed the unpleasantness and the copious evidence of their disregard for me. Especially during my college years as my impaired health made my life more difficult, I was unwilling to relinquish the imaginary emotional support I got from them.

Over the next year and a half, I continually assessed whether or not I was ready to go back to Harvard. Finally, I decided to move back but to live off campus, not in a dorm. I had struggled so much with sleep disruption while living on campus that I was desperate to live in a quiet place. I was lucky to find a rent-controlled sublet through an acquaintance, and I took the train back to Boston with my worldly goods in a few suitcases, ready to build a new life again.

As had been the case since I moved out of the family home when I was fifteen, I avoided asking Dad for money because such requests resulted in unpleasant recriminations and drama. When I first made plans to return to school, Dad told me he would pay my tuition but not my living expenses. He justified this change from our earlier arrangement, in which he had also paid my room and board, by accusing me of arrogance and will-fulness. I thought I could support myself but knew that rent would be expensive, so money loomed large in my mind. The details of "who paid what when" are important because of later events in our family history, and I can rely on the letters I wrote to my grandmother, as well as my journal, for the truth.

As school started that fall of 1982, right after my twentieth birthday, I wrote to my grandmother and put a positive spin on a new waitressing job:

> *Four nights a week should give me enough to live on and pay for books so, for as long as I last there, I won't have to ask for money from Mom and Dad. It will take up a lot of time, but it will also give me a break from studying, and the other girls that work there I think I could like a whole lot.*

Later in the same letter:

*I'm having trouble with Dad because he isn't being straight-forward with me. First he tells me that the family is in severe financial shape, then he tells me that decisions such as what courses I take or whether or not I live on campus are too luxurious for me to make. What he is really saying is that if I don't lead my life exactly as he designates, he won't send me any money. The family is not in severe financial shape. I refuse to believe that it is when he went to Europe and to Guatemala this past summer and bought bronzes and textiles. Also, I have not been in school for a year and a half, during which time I received no money from them. Also, I am leading my life in a moral, responsible way, and I can't imagine how I could lead it any differently that would make him satisfied. The only conclusion I can come to is that he is impossible.*

Dad never provided any guidance on courses or careers. He said I was self-indulgent to take whatever courses I wanted but didn't tell me what courses he thought I should take.

A couple of months into the school year, I wrote to my grandmother again and apologized for the intensity of the previous letter:

*Everything is going very well with me. Dad and I resolved things somewhat, and he is sending me money for rent and food so I quit my waitressing job. The job simply would not have worked out with school. My school schedule right now is very heavy. I'm in class about nineteen hours a week, not including outside assignments and reading.*

Dad had come around and agreed to send me the amount that Harvard charged for room and board, even though my actual expenses for rent and food were a bit higher. He said he would pay the tuition bill directly to Harvard. Sometimes he paid me late or paid me smaller amounts than we had agreed to, and once he "forgot" to pay Harvard, making me register late for classes that term. But, in broad strokes, this was the arrangement that continued over the next few years as I finished school. I did not receive any other money from my parents toward expenses then or in future years. Although I left that waitressing job because it was full-time, I was never unemployed. I preferred food service because of the free meals. In my journal, I wrote:

*estimate expenses:*

| | |
|---|---|
| *$210* | *rent* |
| *25* | *phone and power* |
| *100* | *food* |
| *60* | *dance and bus* |
| *$400* | *a month* |

The following fall I became ill again, this time seriously enough that I left school partway through the term. I was weak and needed to sleep fourteen hours or more most days. I lost about twenty pounds over a period of a few months. I dragged myself to my job because I needed to pay expenses, but I didn't write in my journal or to my grandmother during this time. Today I have no memory of what the trigger for the illness might have been, and in fact that fall is a blank for me. At the time, I tentatively attributed my collapse to depression or a delayed reaction to earlier stresses in my life, but it must have been a chemical reinjury. I just don't remember my environmental circumstances sufficiently to identify the exact cause. Harvard

charged me partial tuition for the interrupted term, which was
$1,200 that I needed to make up to Dad.

I went back to school the next semester but took a light
course schedule because I still felt tired and ill. I started to sprin-
kle pass-fail courses into the lineup to lighten my load and help
me get through the remaining three semesters. From all the
promise it held for me a few years before, Harvard had become
a painful grind. Because I was ill so much and because I worked
so many hours, I never had the chance to develop either the
friendships such a special place can provide or the full intellectual life I had dreamed of.

Today, YouTube videos and Wikipedia list for me the traits of a
psychopath, a sociopath, or a pathological narcissist, but when I
was young I would have just said "creep." Today, I sketch out a
grid with family members at the top and behaviors at the side, and,
running down the lists, I see that an anti-fairy dusting of these
nasty behaviors was sprinkled all over my family.  My brother,
Hunter, and I got the lightest coatings, and my father got the
heaviest by far. It makes sense to me that his seething and fer-
menting mind would have addressed his own childhood trauma
and alienation with not one but two antisocial pathologies, and for
him I can tick all of the boxes for both sociopathy and narcissism.
I see now that he also struggled with bouts of deep depression,
some lasting many years. I'm still under the spell of his beauty and
magnetism and my memories of our early happy years as a family,
but at the same time I wish I had been able to see him clearly and
get him out of my life earlier than I did.

My parents did me a terrible disservice in how they handled
my repeated illnesses while I was in college. When I first left

school, I conjectured in my journal that the problem "might be physiological," meaning chemical. I repeatedly referred to the second time I left school as a time of illness, so I did suspect the problem was not in my mind. I was deeply responsible and hardworking and always had been, so Mom and Dad must have known my life upsets were inadvertent. They could have easily afforded the amounts of money that would have given me ease and security instead of my continual financial anxiety. During these years, Dad traveled frequently and continued to build his collections, indications that he had plenty of cash. He bragged to me often about the weight and success of his various investments in art and real estate. I needed help and support from these two people, but they willfully ignored the overwhelming evidence that I was ill. Instead, by making me bear the financial burdens of these life transitions and by the way they talked to me about my decisions and life circumstances, they recast my misfortunes as my own fault. The worse they treated me, the worse they had to treat me the next time to stick to their story. They were like two rats that are stuck in a stinking dirt hole over a septic field looking at each other questioningly, nodding at the same time, and then keeping on digging.

My parents visited for my graduation. Mom bought me a strange plaid winter coat at a discount store, but I have no memory of any other graduation present from them. In the snapshots, I am thin and wan, with no makeup and bad hair. Under the ceremonial robe, you can see a sweatshirt with the neckband cut out, not a nice dress or blouse. I was worn out. I had tried so hard to make my college experience all that it could be and had been deeply disappointed. Since I was graduating two years after my original class and had lived off campus, I knew almost no one at the ceremony. I had a boyfriend and a few other friends who were at a couple of meals with Mom and

Dad, but I sensed that my parents judged my social life a failure. They acted disapproving and as though they were fulfilling an unpleasant obligation.

Around the time of my graduation from Harvard in 1985, even as I still wanted to be close to them, I started to wonder if perhaps my parents didn't wish me well. It was possible I would not be able to be a success in life, and in their fundamental selfishness they did not want to be responsible for someone who was truly in need. I started to have occasional moments of clarity, during which I understood that my father was a toxic and destructive person whom I should try to eliminate from my life.

# Chapter 18 - The Snapshots

For a few years after college, I was in better shape. I had always loved everything about waitressing, and initially I had no vision for a professional career. I moved from one waitressing job to the next better one and started taking part-time computer science courses. Then, I got progressively better jobs working with computers. I met future Husband, and we were happy together. My health improved a bit, and although I still struggled with fatigue, bad sleep, and menstrual pain, these conditions were not as acute as they had been in earlier years. Mom and Dad sold the apartment building, ironically to my ex-lover Bill, and moved into a house that didn't have rooms set aside for children. When I visited Hometown once a year or so, I stayed with Amy and her boyfriend in their apartment.

Mom and I corresponded by letter and occasionally talked on the phone. She wrote to me on pretty note cards that she bought in museum shops and provided chit-chatty news about her work, travels to see her sisters, her exercise routine. Once for about six months, these cards were unusually frequent, and here I see the hand of her therapist, Bruce. "Think long term," I imagine him advising her as they started this brief reconciliation-lite project together. Then a false reassurance, "You can build whatever kind of relationship with her that you want."

I received a strange phone call from Mom around this time. She stated that she was trying to resolve for herself why the two of us weren't close, but then segued quickly into vague recriminations. She repeatedly told me, "You are exactly like your father." It was broadly acknowledged within our family that Dad was an unreasonable jerk, so saying I was like him wasn't a compliment. Then she went on for a while about how there were two types of people in the world: First, there were those enlightened individuals such as herself and almost everyone else she knew, who knew the glass was half-full and were capable of seeing shades of gray. Then, there were those negative types like me and Dad, for whom the glass would always be half-empty, who were only capable of interpreting the world in terms of black and white.

There were long silences on her side as we both tried unsuccessfully to find anything specific I had done to cause distance between us. Bizarrely, I suggested one reason she and I weren't close was that, unlike Kirsten, I wasn't good at asking her for money. Finally the call ended, and I felt hurt and mystified. I was able to partly discount her comments by articulating to myself that she who only saw two types of people in the world was the one who saw the world in black and white, not me. Now I know that of course it was Bruce who suggested she call me to try to get to a place she felt better about. But when she had me on the phone, all she wanted to do was recast our history, and all she managed to do was insult me repeatedly.

A suspiciously short time after this call from Mom, I had a similarly strange call from Kirsten. Kirsten didn't pretend she had any goal other than to vent and make me feel rotten. She went on and on about what a jerk and an asshole I was. I was just like Dad, was the most selfish person she knew, lacked moral fiber, and didn't treat other people well. Just as I had during the call with Mom, I kept thinking that Kirsten and I had a relationship we could preserve. We didn't talk often, but she was important to me. I tried to understand where she was coming from, so the call lasted longer than I should have allowed it to. Toward the end, I was able to separate myself from her process and watch what she was doing. I knew that when Kirsten berated me because she felt bad inside, she was the one channeling Dad, not me, and I knew what she was doing was unjustified and maybe even unforgivable.

I hadn't spent significant time with either of these people in almost ten years, so they hardly knew me. Probably Kirsten's vitriol was extreme because my earlier call with Mom had made Mom feel bad about herself.

One of my computer jobs was in a newer-construction building, and I became ill with bad sleep, unspecific anxiety, trouble finding words, and trouble concentrating. I was unable to respond with genuine smiles and cheerfulness to my colleagues. I made mistakes in my work, which mystified me because I was usually a careful worker. My boss became unhappy with me, and I was laid off. I blamed her since she was neurotic and uptight, dusted myself off, and got another job.

During these years as when I was a teenager, Dad was rude and dismissive toward me for no apparent reason. I told myself that it was just his thing. At a deeper level, I knew he acted this way because he was caught up with my beauty and was jealous that I had gone to Harvard. I avoided lengthy contact with him, and we did not correspond. I have few letters from him from any period of my life. During early 1987, he came through Boston on a business trip and went out to dinner with future Husband and me. At the restaurant and later at our apartment, Dad was agitated and uncomfortable. He wriggled in his chair and made strange, contorted faces as he talked nonstop about his own interests and activities. I was used to this, but future Husband thought he was a neurotic freak. Now I think he behaved so oddly because he saw that future Husband was a person of weight and integrity and the contrast with his own inner self made him miserable. Dad saw that this man could help me become a different person than the one that he and Mom defined to each other, which is what ended up happening.

Mom and Dad were helping Kirsten pay for law school, and I asked Mom if she would pay for my health insurance while I finished a certificate program in computer science. She turned me down without an explanation. I was disappointed that she supported Kirsten's advanced studies but thought mine were unworthy. Neither Mom nor Dad had ever been explicit about what help they would provide for graduate studies, and I assumed from her turning me down that the answer was "none."

I traveled to Hometown again for the Christmas of 1987 and again stayed with Amy and her boyfriend, visiting my parents' house only a couple of times. Future Husband had agreed to help me duplicate some of the treasured family snapshots that my parents kept in a large shoebox in their house. I planned to make numerous copies of key images so that all the children could have them, and I had discussed my plans with other family members including Mom and Dad. Early during a visit on that Christmas day, after I retrieved the shoebox of snapshots and started looking through them, Dad became upset. Something about the way I got the box down and started flipping through stacks of photos triggered an outburst from him. In an unpleasant scene within earshot of the other gathered family members, he accused me of intending to steal the pictures and also of stealing from him and Mom generally. He indicated that I was not welcome in their house. I felt angry and humiliated, left, and didn't return.

I have never stolen anything from either of them. I have few things they have given me. From Mom, I have a wooden hairbrush, a broken silver barrette, a pair of scissors, and some undistinguished earrings. From Dad, I have photos and negatives that he sent me much later, the infamous and contested omelet pan, two weird rings made of jade, some random antique glass beads, and an antique watch chain I wore as a necklace that he said I could borrow only, not keep, because it was gold. Dad became convinced I was stealing from him and Mom because I deserved so much more than they were willing to give. His broken mind invented theft as the solution to the enormous injustice between them and me.

Dad wrote to me a few days later. Like the other letters of his that I quote in this memoir, I possess the piece of paper he sent me, but I do not own the copyright to his words. I can only quote his letter in part:

> *I believe I must apologize for my behavior while you were in [Hometown] over the holidays. We were, alas, a lot less comfortable together than we were last year at Christmas and when we were together in March in Boston. I write this letter as an effort to assure you that you will always be welcome at our house and to express my sorrow and anger at my own ineptness.*
>
> *For you were not unkind to me and were graceful. What caused my coldness and lack of warmth was a fear that you would be mean to me. There were no upheavals. In the light of what was going on, you were rather forbearing. I am bitter at myself that I could not reveal more openly my happiness in having you among us. I hope I can be less clumsy when we meet again.*

Amy had told him how angry I was, and he realized he had been called out for appalling behavior. To his credit, he apologized and acknowledged my own tempered response. But then he says other family visits were happy and successful times in our lives together, when in fact they were unsatisfactory. He said I would always be welcome in their house when I hadn't been welcome in their home since I was fifteen. He recast his excessive response as motivated by the fear that I would be mean to him, when I had never been unkind to him in any way.

After the disastrous visit and disconcerting letter of apology, I was finally and utterly finished with him and the way he treated me. I knew that he felt connected to me and that I mattered to him, but at last I saw clearly that when he looked at me, he was unable to achieve generosity or kindness. This had been true for as long as I could remember. I started to make plans to offload my father. I would need to get out of the family partnership and trust arrangement that he had set up about ten years before.

# Chapter 19 - The Worm Turns

When Dad established the family partnership and transferred most of the ownership of the apartment building to his children, he told us the assets would be ours when we turned twenty-one, meaning 1983 for me. This did not happen. The apartment building had been sold and turned to cash, and all of the children were at least twenty-one years old, but there was no final accounting and distribution of assets to the children. Although the partnership agreement specified regular reporting on income, expenses, and asset balances, the reporting I got was skimpy and irregular. It showed large movements of cash out of my share during years I was not receiving money for college tuition or anything else. Although the income was taxed at our lower rates, I at least never received it. Whatever Dad's original intentions, the partnership and trust arrangement was now just a giant tax wheeze and cash bucket for him.

I wanted to be rid of him, but that meant becoming more involved while I extricated myself from the partnership. Still angry over his recent treatment of me, I planned to use the opportunity to express my disrespect repeatedly. I wrote several letters to him and to his lawyer indicating that, per the partnership agreement, I had the right to withdraw and receive my asset balance, and this was what they were obligated to do. Each letter gave me a rebellious and self-righteous thrill. Dad ignored me for a while, and then he and Mom sent a letter that was written in her handwriting. The letter began by claiming that they had only recently learned from their lawyer about my requests to withdraw, an obvious untruth since I had written to both Dad and his lawyer directly many times. The letter continued:

> *We want this activity on your part to stop. We remain firm in our conviction that when your undergraduate education was finished we had no further financial obligation to you. We will isolate ourselves from you for several months until we are certain that no further action of this sort has taken place.*

I pressed on and got a lawyer in Hometown, who started corresponding with Dad's lawyer. Dad dug in his heels, and it became clear from the obfuscating tone of his correspondence that he was trying to wear me down until I ran out of cash to pay my lawyer. I don't know what he thought the ultimate resolution would be. It was clear from all the legal documents that I had an absolute right to withdraw if I wanted to, but his authority had been challenged and he took it badly.

The concoctions that Dad and his lawyer put together are outrageous and would be funny if they weren't so obviously designed to intimidate me. Dad's first formal written request for information included, "8. State whether Plaintiff is receiving any psychiatric or medical treatment, the name and address of the physician treating and a summary of the treatment undergone in the last nine (9) years. 9. State when the last time Plaintiff visited her parents. 10. State whether Plaintiff is living with anyone at this time and the relationship of Plaintiff to that individual or individuals."

Then, about a year and a half after the disastrous visit to their house for Christmas, I got a letter from Dad in which he hinted darkly:

*Neither of us expected that things would ever get to this point. Long ago I told [my lawyer] that our object was to get you to stop. You have not stopped and a great deal of damage has occurred. Much worse may be ahead. There are some things that you should know. I am assuming that you understand now what our position would be when and if your mother and I and others are in court. Most of these issues, which have indeed always been on our mind, are better left within the family.*

He meant that if I didn't back down, he and Mom would reveal to the world I was emotionally unstable. This seemed a weak and pointless threat. He tried to bully me through peer pressure:

*The legal fees I am paying are coming from the partnership and trust. That means that Kirsten, Hunter, and Amy and indeed you and I are paying these expenses in equal shares. Your brother and sisters know this.*

This didn't make sense because for many years he had been treating all of the money as his. How could my one-fifth portion of his legal fees be costing me anything if I was never going to get the assets?

He went on to brag about how large his estate was and to threaten to exclude me from it. Then:

*All of us are firm in our opposition to giving you everything
you demand—most particularly at this time and under
the circumstances that have developed. We all want this to
stop. I write you to learn if you might accept some partial
settlement in return for releases, legal guarantees, that you
would not approach your mother and me regarding money
for a convalescent period of time—say five years. We could
then put aside the potentially damaging exploitation that I,
particularly, devoted much of my life as a father to guard
you against. The whole prospect of redoing my will could
be delayed. We all could try (we are eager to do so) again (I
recall warmly your constructive visits here in August and
December of 1986 and my pleasant visit in Cambridge in
the following March) to reintegrate you into the family.*

He provided some news about family members and then
some self-aggrandizing news about himself, including bragging
about planting unusual trees like persimmons and pawpaws. He
wrote some more about how earlier visits had been happy. Then:

*Please do be assured that all of us want you back loving and
laughing and listening to music with us again. I am eager
to hear any proposals you have for making things better.
I repeat my offer to go with you to a psychotherapist in
Boston. There are specialists here now who deal in family
arbitration. If you wish to remain estranged and to consider
only a temporary financial and legal arrangement, perhaps
you could send [future Husband with name misspelled] as
an intermediary.*

This letter contained so many lies that I could not even
consider its request for mediation because I was paralyzed by

the unreality of its contents. I knew that although I had vague health troubles, I was not emotionally unstable as he repeatedly implied. He said that there was some potentially damaging exploitation that he had devoted himself to guarding me against, but this makes no sense at all. Did he mean financial exploitation of me by a boyfriend? I had little money. Sexual exploitation by a boyfriend? I had a normal relationship with future Husband. Was he letting slip that he had always to guard against sexually exploiting me himself? I see now, finally, that my parents must have propagated a myth to each other that I was susceptible to sexual exploitation, as a cover for Dad's leching after me. Yikes.

He painted a picture of a happy family life, but that was a complete lie—the family had not been happy in twenty years. He suggested that I was recently part of the family, but I had not been part of the family since before he and Mom kicked me out when I was fifteen. He said the family wanted me back, but I deeply understood that he, Mom, and Kirsten did not want me to be part of the family. He said he had offered to see a psychotherapist with me, but this was a lie. At the end, he misspelled future Husband's name!

At the time of this letter, I was twenty-six years old. I had undertaken a messy and expensive process to separate myself permanently from my parents, especially my father, because of many years of abuse and neglect. I continued to suffer from a poorly understood and undiagnosed neurological weakness that periodically made me quite ill in ways that were deeply upsetting. I was struggling to support my share of the household with future Husband while some of my workplaces made me ill. Even as I wanted to be free of my father, he was capable of frightening me and hurting me. There is a phrase that has entered the collective consciousness that speaks to the difficulty of resolving emotional trauma when actual events are denied.

Instead, an alternate reality is presented that recasts abusers as well-intentioned and well-behaved. The term is gaslighting, and this is what my father was doing in his letter.

Dad was right about one thing, though. The situation did get worse.

He and his lawyer insisted I travel to Hometown for a deposition, in which we would each be interviewed by the other's lawyer as preparation for a trial. The transcripts from these interviews, which occurred in October of 1989, as well as my memories of my mother and father that day, are my anti-gaslighting weapons.

# Chapter 20 - Deposition

In my quest to separate myself financially from my father and hopefully also put a sharp stick in his eye, I pressed on with the nuclear option. I traveled alone to Hometown for the deposition. I was interviewed by Dad's lawyer with Mom and Dad present, and then Dad was interviewed by my lawyer, whom I'll call Mr. Whitman, with me and Mom present. One of my strongest visual memories of the day was Mom's face, which was like a death mask, colorless and grim. Dad and I greeted each other from across the room, but she was unable to respond to my "Hi, Mom" and instead looked at me throughout the proceedings as though she wanted me to die.

Dad's lawyer asked me about the different places I had lived, my job history from the beginning, how much money I had made at each of the jobs, and how long I'd stayed. He asked me questions about future Husband, such as: how old he was, his job history, his recent salary history and other income, and our monthly expenses and their allocation; also his race, where his father was from, and what his father did for a living. He asked how much money I had and how much money I had when I graduated from college. He asked me about my history of seeing a psychologist or therapist, which was minimal. I felt they were searching for evidence of bad life choices, but there was no such evidence. There was a fairly normal progression of increasing income and job responsibility, minimal participation from the therapeutic profession, and a long-term relationship with an accomplished man. I found these questions invasive and slightly abusive, as though Dad's lawyer had seen too many courtroom dramas in which witnesses are intimidated into capitulation by loud and obnoxious interruptions. I remained absolutely calm and self-assured. He asked me why I had brought the suit:

*[All deposition extracts are unedited except to correct name spellings and add an occasional observation about someone's body language or tone of voice.]*

**A:** . . . that one of the reasons why I brought the suit was to make a statement that I was not willing to be exploited for tax fraud, or whatever other purposes that may have been going on.

**Q:** Exploited for tax fraud?

**A:** Well, exploited. If it turns out that my parents never meant for me to get the money, then clearly they had some other reason for making this arrangement, and one of my conjectures is that it may have been done to evade income taxes.

**Q:** Now, maybe I misunderstood your testimony, but I thought you said that your Harvard education had been paid for out of this trust?

**A:** That's right; it had.

**Q:** And yet you're saying that you believe now that your mother and father never intended for you to get the money?

**A:** No; I think that they may have changed their mind at some point.

**Q:** I see. So—

**A:** I think they may have thought so originally, but then later on decided they would rather keep it themselves; but I really don't know what they think.

**Q:** You don't really know? *(said in a sarcastic tone)*

**A:** Yes.

**Q:** But you think they might be guilty of tax fraud?

**A:** Well, I think that maybe one of the reasons why they are so reluctant to give me the money now is because they would rather keep it.

**Q:** Do you love your mother and father?

**A:** Yes.

**Q:** Do you have any idea how this is making them feel, for you to say these things and bring a lawsuit against them?

**A:** I really don't know how they feel.

**Q:** Are you telling me now that you don't have any—any idea of how this is making them feel, for you to bring a lawsuit against them over this matter and for you to say that they're guilty of tax fraud? (*said in a sarcastic tone*)

**A:** No; I didn't say that they're guilty of tax fraud. I am sure that—-

**Q:** I didn't ask you that, ma'am. I asked you if you have any feelings inside yourself as to how this is making them feel? Your mother and father are sitting here in the room.

**A:** Yes.

**Q:** You do have?

**A:** I do have some idea.

**Q:** And how do you think it's making them feel?

**A:** Well, I imagine that they might be a little ashamed of the things that they've done and not done, and I imagine also that they might be a little worried about what the Internal Revenue would have to say about it.

**Q:** I see.

**A:** So those two are my idea of—

**Q:** So other than that, those are the feelings that you have? You don't have any feelings of shame or remorse about having brought this lawsuit?

**A:** No; I don't. No.

I'm proud of how I handled myself with this man. I stuck to my guns and successfully projected that I was completely truthful and acting in good faith. I was at ease although under considerable stress, and nothing about my tone of voice or body language suggested that I was anything other than determined.

Dad's lawyer wrapped things up with me, and then my lawyer, Mr. Whitman, interviewed Dad. Dad's testimony was remarkable for the number of terrible lies it contained. I was amazed at the wholesale inventions he concocted about family relationships, family financial history, and the history of the family partnership. I still have trouble absorbing all the lies he told and wonder if he possibly believed some portion of them. Throughout this litany of porkies, my mother sat stone-faced. She knew Dad was speaking in whoppers and distorting our family history in order to cast doubts on me as a person, but she let it happen.

Dad did not present as reliable because he pretended not to understand obvious questions, wriggled in his seat, made strange grimaces, and projected discomfort and agitation. Yet everyone except me knew that almost every adjudicating body in the South would believe the testimony of an older white man, whatever his apparent degree of neurosis, over that of a young woman who was living with a biracial boyfriend. Even I became aware as the afternoon wore on that his lawyer was relying on a strong cultural bias that would act to my disadvantage. I intuited this from the nature and tone of the proceedings and also as an unspoken assumption between the lawyers, who seemed a bit too chummy for my liking. In addition to becoming tired from the interrogation, with stress-sweat in my armpits that was the stinkiest of my entire life, I lost faith that justice would be served. The legal case was completely clear-cut, and they didn't have a leg to stand on, yet Dad and his lawyer were acting as though they would win. They knew that in their society, no one would support my story because of the demographic profile of my household.

I went home and a short while later received a further blow. Mr. Whitman forwarded formal legal indications that if the case were to proceed to court, Mom, each of my siblings, and also a good friend of mine were ready to testify as to my emotional instability. Possibly Dad was bluffing, but I found this last deeply hurtful and lost my small remaining appetite for further legal process. Dad offered to release me from the partnership and from any related tax obligations that might arise in the future with a settlement paid to me of $17,000. This amount, which was within spitting distance of my actual expenditures of $15,000, seemed arbitrary at the time. Now I see that most likely Dad's lawyer asked mine how much I had spent so that Dad would know the minimum he could get away with. I accepted and the thing was done.

I never saw my mother or father again. No one in my family attended my wedding, which was small and took place not long after the lawsuit was resolved, nor did I attend any of my siblings' weddings. Once many years later I talked to my mother briefly by accident when she picked up the phone at my younger sister's house. I was struck by the way she seemed to be speaking to an imaginary person who was not me. She and I exchanged a few letters. I received three letters from Dad over the next thirty years and wrote to him once, shortly before his death.

I wonder what I could have done differently, now that I know the breach was to be permanent. My rage at his behavior over the snapshots was the trigger for the lawsuit, but I had wanted out for years. I resented being exploited for tax evasion and also resented being lied to about the ultimate intended disposition of the underlying assets. I prepared my own tax returns, which were complex, and I had to prepare returns in multiple states, all of which annoyed me. What would happen when I got married—would my husband be linked to this mess? I didn't trust Dad to fully protect me if there were trouble with the tax authorities, even if his own cheating caused the trouble. I suspected him of keeping his children legally attached so that he enjoyed control over their lives and of dangling assets just out of reach to force his children to be deferential to him.

Could I have handled the lawsuit differently? With my current knowledge of legal issues and the business world, I would have been more emphatic about the absolute ridiculousness of Dad's position. I'm not sure this would have changed his response because Dad was spoiling for a fight and relished legal engagements. Several years later, as his mother's executor, he hoovered up her assets and sent "sue me please" notes to all her other intended heirs. Later still he quickly escalated the complexity and drama of legal proceedings when my mother wanted a divorce. In the light of these subsequent events and given his knee-jerk unpleasantness and obfuscation when I sued him, lengthy legal proceedings clearly provided him with pleasurable stimulation.

Could I have sweet-talked my way out of the partnership with gentle assurances that I didn't want any money but wanted to build my own life without the entanglement? Maybe that would have worked if our relationship hadn't already been so damaged. For years, he had tended to take immediate offense at anything I said to him, so there wasn't enough good faith between us to build a nondestructive negotiation process. I would have ended up having to hire a lawyer anyway, not gotten any money to offset legal fees, and for years afterward I would have been burdened with a sense of injustice on top of financial loss. Even now as a mature and wiser woman, I am unable to imagine an alternative scenario in which I could have gotten out of these toxic ties without his taking the fight directly into the gutter.

Thirty years on, the transcript of his deposition is invaluable to me. All I need to do to know that he and Mom colluded to cover up the cause of my neurological damage as an infant is read the amazing and extreme lies my father told in his deposition. These lies prove that my parents' mysterious actions over the entire time of our lives together had one and only one underlying motive: to create an alternative truth to cover up the tragic consequences of their negligence when I was a baby. The volume and bizarre nature of Dad's lies, with Mom sitting beside him occasionally nodding in agreement, only make sense as a desperate effort to shore up their imaginary protective construct in which I was a destructive, ungrateful, and unstable daughter.

# Chapter 21 - So Many Lies

When Dad was interviewed by Mr. Whitman when I filed to withdraw from the family partnership, he told many lies. There was obfuscation, in which he pretended not to understand the question, and there were simple lies. Both of these were primarily intended to obstruct the progress of my lawsuit. There were lies to cover up illegal transfers of funds, meaning to hide his own theft and fraud, and there was denial of historical fact and fabrication for him to appear less of an awful father. Finally, there were lies to perpetuate my parents' mythology about my true nature and behavior. As a gestalt, the lies convey the deep rot at the core of Southern society at that time, in which someone such as he could lie and lie and lie in front of his wife and a passel of lawyers, one of whom was his own lawyer and a long-time close friend, and somehow this behavior was accepted as necessary and excusable.

Here is an example of obfuscation:

**Q:** All right, sir. What was the initial contribution of the trust to the partnership?

**A:** I don't understand that.

**Q:** What did the trust have to contribute to the partnership? Did they have a building, did they have money?

**A:** The trust?

**Q:** You had—your children's trust.

**A:** I think—I still don't understand what you're saying.

**Q:** What went into the children's trust?

**A:** You mean went into—what was the partnership? Went into the partnership?

**Q:** From the trust into the partnership.

**A:** I still don't know what you're saying.

**Q:** OK. Let's take it one at a time. You have the trust, with your wife being the trustee?

**A:** Yes.

**Q:** She was the trustee of certain properties or cash or security or something like that?

**A:** Yes; uh-huh.

**Q:** What was she the trustee over? What items? When the trust was created, what was put into the trust?

**A:** I think you better ask the question so that I can answer it.

**Q:** I don't know how else I can ask it. Did the trust have cash?

**A:** The asset—now, I don't know what you want me to say—the asset was an apartment building.

**Q:** All right; and did the trust contribute all or a portion of their interest in the apartment building to the limited partnership?

**A:** I still don't understand what you are getting to. The asset that we're talking about was an apartment house. I think we—we're agreed on that.

**Q:** Is that—

**A:** OK.

**Q:** Is that what, in fact, generated dollars for the limited partnership?

**A:** Yes.

**Q:** For a period of time, the apartment generated dollars through rents; is that correct?

**A:** Yes.

The simple lies went as follows: he sent financial reporting annually to the children; he offered to lend me money from the partnership to buy a house; he didn't remember if the building was in his name; he didn't remember any time Mom might have signed my name for me; he didn't know why my fiancé's race was brought up when I was deposed; he was wrong when he told me

I was a limited partner rather than a beneficiary of the trust; he didn't know if his intent was to give the assets to the children when they turned twenty-one; he didn't know what his intentions were after the ten-year extension of the trust; he didn't know if he had a choice about the disposition of the assets; he didn't know what his choices would be; he didn't remember writing me a letter telling me that their financial obligations to me were over; he didn't feel he had an obligation to make periodic distributions; he made regular birthday and Christmas distributions to the children; he didn't know if there were ever any distributions made by Mom as trustee to the children; he couldn't remember if a $50,000 loan from the partnership to himself had been repaid; and so on.

Relative to fraud, in the partnership accounts there were two large sets of distributions during the years 1985 and 1986, each marked as distributions to Dad's children. One set went for taxes on the sale of the apartment building in 1985, and the other set, totaling $44,000, was mysterious.

**Q:** Do you recall writing those checks?

**A:** I wrote them.

**Q:** But you don't recall the purpose?

**A:** No. (*said while wiggling and looking uncomfortable in his chair*)

**Q:** Do you know what happened to those funds?

**A:** I don't know.

**Q:** You don't know if they were deposited into one account, endorsed to the IRS, you just don't know?

**A:** I don't know.

**Q:** When did you buy the house where you live now?

**A:** April or May of 1985.

**Q:** Were any of these funds, to your knowledge, utilized in any way to facilitate the purchase of that residence?

**A:** I don't know.

**Q:** Were you aware of the financing on the purchase of your residence?

**A:** Yes.

**Q:** Did you borrow money to buy that residence?

**A:** No.

**Q:** Did you pay cash for the residence?

**A:** Yes.

**Q:** Where did that cash come from?

**A:** I don't remember.

Later Mr. Whitman circled back around to this mysterious set of checks Dad had written, and again Dad said he could not recall what they were for. It was obvious to everyone in the room that Dad had taken the cash to buy his house and noted that the distributions had gone to the children when they had not, not least because of his squirming and gesticulating while he was being questioned about them.

I had indicated to Mr. Whitman that I didn't want to set an ugly tone about our family history, so he didn't press Dad about some of Dad's truly terrible behavior. But some emotive aspects of my family history did come up, and Dad lied about them so that he would appear to have been a less awful father than he was. To my surprise, he and Mom possessed awareness that his true actions would look bad to others.

**Q:** All right. Do you recall when she was fifteen and your older daughter, Kirsten, was seventeen, that they moved into a separate apartment?

**A:** Yes.

**Q:** How did that come about?

**A:** Through a great deal of family turbulence.

**Q:** All right; and, again, was it your request to them to leave the house and move into a separate apartment?

**A:** We decided, my wife and I decided that this would be best for the family.

**Q:** All right; and at that point your two daughters moved into the separate apartment?

**A:** Yes.

**Q:** Correct?

**A:** Yes.

**Q:** Am I also correct that they then bought their own, paid their own utilities, supported themselves?

**A:** That's wrong—no.

**Q:** All right. What did you provide for them when they were in this separate apartment?

**A:** We supported them.

**Q:** Fully?

**A:** Yes. *(said while squirming)*

**Q:** Were either of them working at the time; do you know?

**A:** Pookie was a senior in high school and Kirsten was not. Kirsten was working, yes. That was a mistake; Kirsten was working.

**Q:** All right. Was Pookie working?

**A:** I don't know.

**Q:** Do you recall if, in fact, they were buying their own clothes?

**A:** I don't recall.

**Q:** Do you know if they were paying their own utility bill?

**A:** I don't recall.

**Q:** Do you know if they were purchasing their own food?

**A:** I recall supporting them at that time.

This was a lie. My journal is clear that I was buying my own food and clothing and paying my own telephone bill. My social security wage history indicates that I worked over seven hundred hours that year at the sandwich shop, plus I worked for cash for Dad as janitor in the apartment building. Once Dad made us move apartments because he wanted to renovate alongside us and was done renovating the first one we were living in. It cost my sister and me $30 to have our phone service transferred, and I agonized in my journal about asking Mom or Dad to reimburse us for this charge. My share of this telephone company bill represented several hours of my minimum-wage job.

Dad went on about how good relations had been within the family for many years before I started the action to withdraw from the partnership. This was a lie, as for many years I had not felt welcome in their house and had to tiptoe around his feelings for him not to explode.

He fabricated bizarre events:

**A:** From time to time I would ask a child who had a very high balance to go with me to the bank and cash a large check; and then I would hand the sum, after that money was cashed, to the child who needed it.

**Q:** In cash?

**A:** In cash.

**Q:** How often has that occurred?

**A:** In the case of Pookie, very often.

**Q:** That she would be the recipient of the cash?

**A:** Yes.

**Q:** When you say "very often," could you be more specific?

**A:** I cannot. It happened several times. Let's say it happened several times. And that it was—or I attempted to keep those balances level. A mistake, Mr. Whitman.

**Q:** From whose account would these sums be taken that were given to Pookie?

**A:** Typically, the person who was not going to an expensive university.

**Q:** Do you recall specifically whose accounts were utilized in giving this cash to you?

**A:** Mostly Hunter and Amy.

**Q:** Do you recall the amounts that you're talking about?

**A:** I can't recall specifically, but it would be somewhere from four to seven thousand dollars at a time.

**Q:** Over the life of the trust?

**A:** No; each time.

**Q:** Each time?

**A:** Uh-huh.

**Q:** How many times?

**A:** I don't know.

**Q:** You don't recall how many times you distributed between four and seven thousand dollars cash to her?

**A:** No; I don't.

**Q:** Was it more than ten times?

**A:** I don't know.

What he was describing never happened. Mr. Whitman asked him about these events again later, and Dad stuck to his story.

**Q:** You indicated earlier that one of the children would accompany you to the bank and make a withdrawal. Would you go through the mechanics of that for me again?

**A:** Well, we would go to the bank. I would write a check with them. We would go to the bank; they would cash it. They would hand me an envelope with the cash in it; then I would give it to the person that needed it.

**Q:** All right; so you would write a check to them?

**A:** Yes.

**Q:** They would endorse it?

**A:** Yes.

**Q:** And then they would give the cash to you?

**A:** And then I would hand it on.

At the time of the deposition I was mystified by this story, but I have since figured out the reason for it. Mom and Dad worried that if I requested copies of actual checks written from the partnership accounts, the records would reveal that their support during my college years was bare-bones. They invented a scenario whereby I had been given large amounts of cash in addition to actual checks written to Harvard for tuition or to me for rent and food. Possibly Dad did write checks to Hunter and Amy that they then cashed and handed back to him. If so, because the story was partly true, he figured I would have trouble proving that I had not been given the cash. The boldness of this lie speaks to their disregard for me personally. They didn't care that I knew they were lying since they didn't care about me or what I thought.

Dad blamed me for conflicts about money:

**Q:** Had there ever been any conflict between you and Pookie over finances?

**A:** Many.

**Q:** Many?

**A:** Many.

**Q:** How far back does that go?

**A:** All the way.

**Q:** Tell me what you mean, "all the way"?

**A:** It was the usual—it was the usual. It was about money.

**Q:** I mean, are we talking back to high school days?

**A:** I can't recall that, but I do recall that—I recall it very, very keenly when she started Harvard. And that's—it was about money.

**Q:** Where she would make requests from you for funds, and you would say no?

**A:** You have to state it differently, Mr. Whitman.

**Q:** Well, I'm trying to get from you what the conflicts were. Would she request funds from you?

**A:** She wanted more money—

**Q:** All right.

**A:** —than I gave.

**Q:** All right.

**A:** And that was always the case.

Dad was trying to recreate me as a greedy and unsympathetic person. Then he took things further and said he was afraid of physical violence from me.

**Q:** We spent a great deal of time talking about Pookie having counseling, Pookie changing jobs, Pookie taking some time away from school. Are you concerned about your daughter's mental capacity or emotional state?

**A:** Yes.

**Q:** What are your concerns?

**A:** I love my daughter.

**Q:** Do you feel that she's operating under some disability at this time?

**A:** Yes.

**Q:** What disability?

**A:** She is causing damage to far too many people because of money.

**Q:** But do you feel that she is an intelligent girl?

**A:** Yes.

**Q:** Do you feel that she is able to provide for herself?

**A:** Yes.

**Q:** Is she able to live on her own, in your opinion?

**A:** Yes.

**Q:** Do you see her as a threat to herself or anyone else?

**A:** Yes.

**Q:** Who do you see her as a threat to?

**A:** Her mother and me.

**Q:** You're not concerned that physically she's going to do anything to you, are you?

**A:** It has to do with love, Mr. Whitman.

**Q:** All right; but you're not suggesting that she would be doing anything violent to herself or anyone else, are you?

**A:** At this time, no.

**Q:** All right. What do you mean, "at this time"?

**A:** It's been on my mind many times before.

**Q:** Has she ever been a violent person?

**A:** Yes.

**Q:** All right; when was that?

**A:** Arguments at home.

**Q:** Anything physical?

**A:** Yes.

**Q:** When was that?

**A:** These are details I think I'd rather not recall, but I should say that these are the foundation for our concerns.

**Q:** All right; what are we talking about? When she was how old?

**A:** The age of fifteen onwards.

**Q:** Would that have been around the time that you asked her to move out of your apartment and move into a separate apartment?

**A:** Yes.

This is a ghastly and terrible lie. I was never violent toward anyone in my family and instead was meek and oddly well-behaved. I taught my parakeet to talk, cleaned the bathroom weekly, propagated houseplants, was in high demand as a babysitter, was a teacher's pet, and worked in an ice cream parlor and sandwich shop. Jeepers.

I was worn down and frightened by the lies that Dad told in this deposition. I was also unsettled and saddened by the looks on my parents' faces that day. I knew I had to get these people away from me, but at the time I could not fully process everything I learned. Many of the messages I am only now receiving. Only now do I understand that they created a false family history to cover up the worst mistake of their own lives, which was to inadvertently destroy my neurological and chemical resilience when I was an infant and then lie about how it had happened. Because they never told me about the damage, I wasn't able to develop practical approaches for limiting reinjury. Instead, my parents witnessed the repeated impairments I suffered as I grew up, went to college, and got jobs as a young adult. They were desperate to rewrite the past and also to shed responsibility for me. Their solution was to blame me for my own condition by creating a false, unattractive and destructive personality with vaguely defined emotional instability, instead of the real me.

Dad's lies were excessive and gratuitous because he wanted to take full advantage of this chance to codify their fake history. If he swore it was the truth in a deposition, then their version of our story would stand a better chance of being believed in the future. This was why he forced me to travel to Hometown for the legal proceeding. I have the documentary proof of the real events in my journal and letters from those years, so I can reinterpret his lies and reveal their true purpose.

# Chapter 22 - Trouble at Jobs

While the lawsuit proceeded and in subsequent years, I worked in office spaces that caused me fatigue, bad sleep, trouble connecting with colleagues, and a vague sense that life was more of a struggle than it should have been. Then I got a job in a brand-new building at a software company, and this workspace affected me more strongly. I had terrible trouble sleeping at night and also terrible trouble understanding the work I needed to do. I would nod off in my office and have to put my head on my desk. I had trouble staying awake even in meetings and worried about being fired. I had trouble chewing and swallowing, with food and drink often causing coughing fits because they went down the wrong way. I accidentally bit the inside of my mouth a lot. There was an episode where a friend at work told me she was leaving for another job, and I said things to her along the lines of "Fuck you." I had entered some mental state where I wasn't myself and had no control over what I said or did. Our friendship evaporated, and for many years I felt shame every time I remembered that conversation. Shortly after this fugue-state episode with my unlucky friend and due to my deep discomfort in the workplace, I left that job. The building had been constructed from materials that were making me sick.

Looking back at this particular job especially, I marvel that no one around me realized it was a medical issue. But the symptoms were easily interpreted as psychological for the most part. Also, my parents had told me I had a bad character and destructive intentions. I didn't believe them completely, but I did acknowledge that there was evidence of some undefinable mental weakness. I had in the past been to see two therapists for short periods of time but hadn't gotten any benefit from the visits. Now I see this was because the problems were not psychological. Because the damage was neurological, I was impaired and not able to assess my own condition. My work ethic made me knuckle down, grit it out, and do the best job I could for whoever was paying my salary, instead of stepping back to assess my own health situation with clarity.

I had been pursuing a career in computers for about seven years at that point, but I felt financial insecurity because of my checkered job history. I wanted training in a more versatile and high-demand craft to help me get through any future health upsets, so I made plans to go back to school to study accounting.

Around this time, some years after the resolution of the lawsuit, I got a letter from Dad, the first contact between us since the lawsuit. He wrote about a tree the two of us had planted together near the apartment building and bragged that he regularly snuck over in the early morning darkness to prune and fertilize it. This seems extremely unlikely to me because evergreens of the type he and I planted usually require neither pruning nor fertilizer. Then he wrote:

> *This tree is but one of the constant reminders of my love and ineradicable concern for you. There are other reminders. Looking through our carrousels of slides and other pictures taken on trips or festive occasions provides vivid recollections*

*of the happiness you reveled in and inspired in the family. Any of the many interludes of family nostalgia necessarily brings with it reminders of you and our enduring affection as well as our lamentations and regrets.*

He wrote about wanting me at his side to revel in new things in the family's lives and bragged *again* about his eccentric gardening using persimmons, pawpaws, hybrid chestnuts, and oriental pears. He wrote:

*Your mother hovers over her vegetable garden and tends the sprawling iris beds that came with the house. We have purchased (yes, you guessed it!) a rundown property on an acre of neglected (right again!) land. Hunter and I have cleared the place and are putting in massive plantings that will surely become splendid in the coming years. The fantasies have you at our sides wittily commenting on our successes and rejoicing in them.*

Oddly, in a previous letter from a few years earlier, before the lawsuit, he said that their new house sat on a half acre, not a full acre. Also, I had visited this house. It was where he accused me of stealing snapshots. When I was there, I found both the house and the yard to be tidy and not romantically run-down at all. He continued:

*In the nostalgic waves that ever more accompany me as I age, I have concluded that I was happiest as a young father. And many of my happiest moments as a young father were when I was with you—amazed, gratified at your growing beauty and brilliance. This letter is, of course, an appeal for a reconciliation. It is, more specifically, an appeal for you to express to us that you want some sort, almost any sort, of alleviation of our estrangement. If you have suggestions, I yearn, pray for them. I have specific as well as vague notions as to what we might start to do to make things better. But I would like very much first to hear from you that proposals from us would be accepted and pondered—that much of the happiness in our past is not irretrievably lost—that our enduring love may spiritually nourish all of us again and forever.*

This letter gave me the creeps when I first read it, and it still gives me the creeps. His descriptive images did not accurately reflect our time together. Back then I was not aware of the secret burdens my parents felt when they looked at me, but I did know my father didn't care about my happiness. I also knew I didn't give a shite about his pawpaw trees.

Knowing what I now know about my parents' cover-up of the cause of my illness, I'm not sure why he made this play to be in touch again. Possibly he got pleasure from rereading his own honeyed words—he and I have that in common. Maybe because he and Mom had gotten away with the big lie about my illness for so many years, and he became confused by the cumulative tangle of lies and thought he would get away with all of the deposition lies as well. Probably this letter from an apparently loving father had a secondary intended audience, namely other members of the family.

Maybe he assumed I would return to my previous role within the family as cheerful, ignorant dupe. Power isn't much fun if there isn't a serf to shit on. As an extreme narcissist, he was unhappy being ignored and wanted to loop me back into his circle of influence, to have me paying court again, tiptoeing around his feelings and listening to his complaints in return for future largesse (which never arrived!). He was trying to get the abuse-and-apology cycle going again. For me this overwrought and gaslighting letter was a further blast of vomitosis, a forceful expulsion of vile-smelling chunky liquid in my direction in the form of more lies, lies, lies. I had been dumped at the crossroads to hell, and I turned away and did not write him back.

I was around thirty when, in pursuit of enhanced career resilience, I attended a masters-level program in accounting that also awarded an MBA. I graduated first in my class with all A's and one A-minus while working twenty hours a week as a teacher's assistant and research assistant. I put the last semester's tuition on a credit card and sat for the CPA exam, which I passed the first time with scores in the nineties on three of the four sections. I made this extraordinary effort because after my earlier career disruptions I wanted to prove there wasn't anything wrong with me and that I was an accomplished and worthy person.

I was at my first accounting job, at the company now known as PricewaterhouseCoopers (PwC), for four and a half years. Toward the end of that time, there was renovation going on in my workspace. People were painting walls and working with joint compound and other construction materials nearby. There was a lot of construction dust. I started having much more trouble sleeping and would wake up in the middle of the night with what felt like an anxiety attack or a seizure. I felt malaise and had trouble concentrating at work. I put my head down on the desk frequently and got nasty adrenalin shocks when there was noise in neighboring cubes. I had trouble connecting and communicating with people at work, and friendships I had made deteriorated. I did associate my ill health with the construction going on, but I didn't get any support from my supervisors. The only solution I could think of was to leave that job.

I took several months off to recover a bit and then got a job at a nonprofit. A little while later I was contacted with a job offer from a venture capital firm that had been a client of mine at PwC. I knew these people well, they appreciated what I could do for them, and this job offer almost doubled my salary at the nonprofit, so I accepted.

The people at my new job liked me and liked my work. I received gifts of expensive meals and gold jewelry. There were hints that I and a close colleague, who had been there for many years, might receive tiny slivers of interest in upcoming partnership issuances. After several months passed at this job, my office was built out with a new desk, cabinets, and other furnishings. This furniture would have been made with formaldehyde and standard finishes and glues. Immediately I started having terrible health problems. I could not sleep and was deeply uncomfortable with dark thoughts. I became unable to talk cheerfully or even normally to my colleagues in my office environment, where relationships were especially important. By coincidence and at the same time, I had a tumor of unknown severity in one breast that was bleeding continuously through the nipple, our car was breaking down in ways that could not reasonably be fixed, and my husband was having serious health issues of his own. Shortly after my office remodel, I got my period and bled heavily for a week, which was not normal for me. I lost about four times as much blood as usual during that menstrual cycle, on top of all my other health symptoms.

Things came to a head when I had a disagreement with my supervisor, who had just returned from maternity leave after having twins. I don't remember it well. I know I did not say

aggressive or violent things, but I did say weird and socially awk-
ward things. I used inappropriate language, saying "fucking" to
describe some work projects that I truthfully did not mind at all,
and I behaved strangely, with eye contact and facial expressions
that indicated distress. I went home, and when I returned to
the office the next day I was fired. It was evident from the exit
proceedings that my supervisors had spent most of the prior day
talking to their counsel and preparing for my departure.

Even after this debilitating episode, I still didn't understand what was wrong. I thought I had vague psychological
problems that were incapable of proper diagnosis but that probably came from some inherent weakness in my nature, as well
as issues left over from my dysfunctional family. I thought this
underlying weakness had been exacerbated by a string of bad
luck right then in the rest of my life. It is clear to me now that
the new furniture had made me ill, and that my strange words
and actions the day before I was fired came from extreme neurological distress. The neurological and adrenal disruption from
the chemicals in the furniture had also triggered my excessive
menstrual bleeding.

The loss of this particular job and the loss of my professional relationships with these powerful and wealthy people
felt catastrophic to me. I was deeply shaken, ashamed, and disappointed. I also suffered from the longer-term impact of the
neurological reinjury and had depression, bad sleep, unspecific
anxiety, and fatigue for several months. It was the year 2000, and
I was thirty-eight years old. Because Husband was an artist, I
had evolved into the primary breadwinner in our household, yet
despite my academic accomplishments I was seemingly incapable
of normal career progression. I decided I needed to survive as
best I could, shore up my finances against future catastrophes,
and settle for a diminished life in the future.

As I look back on this tale of woes, I know it was my own behavior and my impaired neurological state that repeatedly caused me either to be fired or to become so uncomfortable that I left a job of my own volition. Yet, I do wish I had encountered more basic kindness along the way. My behavior wasn't destructive, aggressive, or violent. It was weird and socially unacceptable in that business world. Each time it only became weird after a while, meaning I had a chance to develop normal professional relationships with people at first. Yet, no one saw that there was something wrong with my health and that I needed help. Even at the venture capital firm, where the halls were loaded up with billionaires who all knew my name and spoke to me in familiar and friendly terms at the beginning, no one was big enough or capable of sufficient basic kindness and generosity to register that I was in trouble. My health nose-dived over a period of a few weeks, and none of my coworkers had sufficient kindly intentions to interpret my behavior as anything other than inconvenient and potentially threatening to themselves.

There is a terrible stigma attached to mental illness, and those who judge have no regard for a person's history, true nature, or intentions. It is deeply hurtful to blame a person who is ill for their illness, even if the primary symptoms are behavioral, cognitive, or both. The competitive nature of our current society, in which decisions and judgments are based on the selfish tenets of the capitalist faith, is destructive to the large numbers of people who have received hidden damage from their toxic environments. The solution is a post-neoliberal, more compassionate approach that recognizes the primary importance of aggregate health instead of money.

Although I had many upsets as well as low-level chronic ill health, the years of my late twenties through my late forties weren't completely bleak. I have always been an approval junkie, so I enjoyed working hard at my jobs, and, if I wasn't ill, I received good performance reviews. I kept myself fit with jogging and lap swimming. Most of the time I was a cheerful and intellectually curious person. During those years, I didn't dress as badly as I do now. Today, I've given up and have fully embraced a scruffiness that is several clicks past casual, but back then I was still trying, tortuously and with intermittent success, to wear appropriate and attractive clothing from day to day. I would buy an article of clothing, not wear it for years while hating it more and more, and finally bring it to Goodwill along with a few other despised and depressing clumps of useless and sad fashion, maybe picking up a few new ones at Goodwill while I was there. I'm not sure why as an adult I have always been terrible at buying clothes—probably for many boring reasons. I didn't look like much outside of the house, but then as now I had the firm conviction and enormous consolation that I looked great naked. Husband and I developed many common interests, including watching British movie and television productions, visiting art museums, and going on road trips. He sings doggerel when he is happy and has always been an avid and accomplished cook, so our home smelled and sounded comforting. I have always felt completely loved by him.

# Chapter 23 - Therapy

About a year ago, I was ill because I was working on sewing projects using recycled sweaters that had mothball residuals in them. I didn't smell anything and had aired out the old sweaters for months and washed them repeatedly. Evidently, they had traces that were imperceptible but still damaging to me. I got gradually worse and worse at the same time that I was lining up doctors' appointments to get documentation in advance of applying for social security disability. When I went in for the appointments, I was genuinely adversely affected and depressed, and my primary care doctor recommended I see a therapist.

I have intermittent anxiety and sometimes feel low from my life's traumas. These become worse when an adverse environmental exposure has undermined my neurological balance. I was feeling roughed up at the time, so on the surface it was reasonable for me to accept this treatment suggestion. Sometimes I worry that I could become so neurologically impaired that I'm unable to properly communicate my need for a fragrance- and chemical-free environment. Because I'm unable to insist on this protection, I am inadvertently made more and more ill. This particular nightmare is perhaps an echo of my initial illness, during which I had no language to express my suffering because I was too young to speak. Whether it is memory or premonition, this experience of mute anguish haunts me regularly. So, when my doctor recommended a therapist, I thought that if I had someone in the medical profession who understood the whole story, they could be an advocate for me in this helpless state. Because my primary care doctor usually held appointments in fifteen-minute blocks, I hoped a local therapist who had an hour at a time to absorb my story would be this person.

Only twice before had I sought help from a therapist. The first time was the semester before I dropped out of college when I was a sophomore. My therapist was in her mid-thirties but still in training, and she was so nervous that she made me ill at ease. Once, just by way of chatting, I asked her what town she lived in. She responded with agitation, as if she believed my casual question about her personal life meant I planned to do her some harm. She was a damaged person who lacked empathy, and I quit after a few sessions with her.

A few years later, around the time I became ill and had to leave college for the second time, my mother paid for me to see a psychologist. This woman was a seasoned professional whose hourly rate was a burden to me, even though my mother was paying. She dressed much like my mother, in understated yet elegant professional attire and minimal makeup. I met with her a few times, during which she said almost nothing to me. Then, my mother came through town on a trip and met with my psychologist for an hour. Afterward both of them seemed to be hiding something important when I separately asked them about their meeting. Probably because Mom was paying, she had managed to co-opt the relationship, just as she had when I met that one time with her therapist Bruce a couple of years earlier. My mother and this woman were demographic peers with similar professional credentials and experience, so my mother was able to use their status as distant colleagues to spin the doctor's perceptions of me. I quit soon after because I didn't like the woman. Among other therapists I know or knew in the past on a personal level, a high proportion are neurotics whom I wouldn't trust to possess basic kindness. Both of my mother's sisters are in the therapeutic profession as is my younger sister, Amy, and, as I said to Husband, I'd rather eat my own scrotum than rely on their ilk for enlightened advice. Despite my reservations, I decided to give therapy a chance again because I did want to shore up my support network within the local medical profession.

My primary care doctor referred me to an agency that provided mental health services to the poor. The offices were in a warren of partially underground rooms in a commercial office building that happened to be close to my house. The waiting room contained a few folks who looked truly down-and-out. The reception area air was heavy with the familiar cocktail of industrial smells in buildings of relatively new construction or renovation that are commercially cleaned. The smell is a result of poor ventilation, fragranced cleaning products, inexpensive carpets and furnishings that are loaded up with formaldehyde and other foam toxins, and off-gassing paint, caulk, and other interior construction materials. I wore my half-face respirator in the waiting room, but for my first visit I didn't wear it in the therapist's office. That room, though underground and windowless, seemed not to smell by comparison, and I wanted a better chance of actually connecting with my therapist, David.

David's office was nicely furnished and scattered with tasteful and subtly colorful decorative objects. I provided family background and talked about my life in broad strokes. By the end of the fifty minutes, I was having trouble finding words and tracking my thoughts, which meant there were airborne

chemicals in the environment that were affecting my neurological state. I explained to David that I would need to wear my
mask in the future, and this was fine with him.

For the second and third weekly visits, we met in his permanent office, as the prior space, he explained, had been borrowed
from a colleague. This room was markedly dreary, with a couple
of brightly colored, fake Georgia O'Keeffe clitoris-type images
and mismatched chairs. I inhaled only through my cartridge
respirator, and the office didn't make me sick. I talked more
about my illness and how it limited everything I did. I told him
that I was struggling to make sense of my relationships with my
parents and my siblings and that I was working toward a full
acceptance that my mother and father knew I had been adversely
affected by the childhood exposure and did not tell me.

David was prone to talking about how trauma affects
the physical nature of the brain. This was not helpful to me. I
wanted true sympathy, validation of my recent insights into my
family history, and practical suggestions on how to craft a new
life. As I explained to him, I wanted a relationship with a local
therapist who would help me if I were ever truly in trouble. We
made progress covering the relevant family history in the first
three meetings but then didn't have a specific plan for next steps.
We agreed to wait an interval of three weeks to meet again.

When we reconvened, apparently David had not reviewed
his notes, because he needed to be reminded of key issues. He
also frequently covered his mouth with his hand. I had brought
in something to show him, and to do this I moved to a seat that
was closer to him without the low table in between us. When I
didn't move back to my original seat, he gradually inched across
the carpet until he was a couple of feet farther away than he had
been at the outset of our conversation. His arms were folded
across his chest. I realized I had started to focus on being polite

to him as a cover for his detachment and the irrelevance of his comments, as if we were at a bad cocktail party. These were not good signs.

Toward the end of our meeting, I asked him about documentation he could provide in case the social security disability determination folks were in touch with him. We agreed it would be relevant that I wore a cartridge respirator during our meetings, and that during the first meeting when I hadn't I had suffered obvious cognitive impairment. A little later he grew cagey about what he would be willing to attest. He referred to *my* reality, implying that this might be different from objective reality. I intuited that he was unwilling to say that he had observed and did believe I had chemical intolerance. He was unwilling to take a stand even though it was all we had talked about for four hours, and during our first meeting he had seen with his own eyes that I deteriorated without my mask.

We agreed to meet again in three weeks, but on reflection I decided the relationship had become pointless. I didn't feel any connection or support, as evidenced by his distancing body language and unwillingness to acknowledge my illness. He was never going to be an advocate if I were in trouble. I offloaded David as a dud.

Why was David unable to help me? Although my history is complex, my issues are simple. I am basically happy and am summoning my deep core of resilience to build an unconventional new life after terrible devastation that was not self-inflicted. I want encouragement and support.

The usual fare for David is people who are messed up because they have made terrible life choices or are making terrible continuing actions not fully of their own volition because of addiction. My story was not in David's playbook. Even professionals in human misery have trouble absorbing how profoundly unlucky I have been. David was lazy, he lacked the curiosity to connect with the complexities of my story even though he was paid to do so, and he was almost certainly impaired by the airborne chemicals in his vile-smelling office space.

The pattern was the same with the two therapists I had seen at least thirty years earlier. Each was a mild parasite and absolutely useless to me. Considering therapists I've known personally and therapists I've seen as a patient, my experience is not deep, but it is broad. The profession is bankrupt, and to a huge degree these people do not provide useful insight or advice.

The fundamental rot at the core of the profession is that psychologists and therapists have been forced to invent behavioral and personality-based explanations and motivations for symptoms that are based in neurology, by which I mean chemistry. They provide erroneous, frankly bullshit explanations for problems that are due to the effects of chemicals on the brain. People need to discern the underlying causes of cognitive and behavioral problems suffered by themselves or their loved ones if visiting a therapist has provided only minimal benefit. The effects these chemicals are having on humanity are pervasive and deeply damaging. Put simply, your fragranced fabric softener is making you stupid and depressed. Your shampoo and hair dye are making you sleep badly. The smells inside your car are making your children unable to concentrate. The off-gassing from computer cables and carpets is making you tired at work. These are not problems that therapy can solve.

Some might say I have mental health issues because when I have had an adverse exposure, I have cognitive and behavioral changes. I have trouble finding words, and I have dark thoughts.

If the exposure has been extreme, I behave strangely and say odd things. But this effect is neurological, not psychological, and there are physical symptoms at the same time, such as terrible sleep, fatigue, noise sensitivity, and seizure-like convulsions in my head. I may have symptoms of depression, but they are based on a physical event, meaning chemical imbalance or damage to my nervous system.

Medical professionals I saw when I became so ill at age forty-eight were unable to understand the distinction between chemically induced mental anguish and distress caused by emotional factors. They referred to both conditions as "depression." I spoke at length about this to my then primary care physician, and she was unable to fathom the difference. Similarly, a cold-hearted and cynical neurologist (Is there one who isn't?) refused to meet me partway when I tried to explain this difference to him. There is a lexical gap, meaning our vocabulary is not adequate to describe neurological distress caused by a chemical event. But the difference is crucial to understand many conditions that current therapy modalities cannot mitigate and to bring these conditions out of the margins and into the mainstream.

We need a phrase to describe a chemical event that affects neurology, or we need to bring a current medical phrase out of obscurity and into wide usage. If I knew Latin, I could come up with a good one, but I will use "chem-ev" for now. The chemical event could be the result of environmental exposure, secondary sensitivity-based disruption like I have, oral ingestion of a neuro-affecting substance, or even hormonal fluctuations. We need a phrase to describe the neurologically impaired state of a person suffering from a chem-ev. Obviously, "depressed" is not the right word. How about "chem-crapped"?

If I have a chem-ev and have both physical and neurological symptoms of chem-crap, therapy will not help me. Once we have language to describe the event and the resulting condition, it is ludicrous to suggest that psychotherapy is the answer. We gain enormous power and can choose more appropriate approaches and treatments for ourselves and our loved ones.

If you restrict your movements and also the goods and foods that you consume, you will be in a better position to observe the effects that your environmental exposures have on your mood, your sleep quality, and other manifestations of your neurological state. You will be able to help your family members and friends get to the bottom of their own medical and behavioral reactions to environmental stimuli. For example, even a tiny exposure to fragranced laundry products makes me sleep badly; how can these products not be affecting people who are practically bathing in the stuff? People with bipolar disorder should do a deep dive into their environmental exposures, diet, and other potential factors, to tease apart the likely triggers for their disrupted state. People with recurrent depression should look closely at the chemicals, fragrances, and foods they ingest and try to discern the underlying pattern, which surely exists. Autism, childhood asthma, childhood behavioral disorders, and many other maladies should be analyzed from this angle. The current medical profession has a bias against making these connections because of peer pressure and because corporations fund so much medical research. We need to think outside the box and make these connections ourselves until we can drag along the doctors, even if they kick.

# Chapter 24 - InsCo

In 2001, a few months after my devastating firing by the board-room full of billionaires and near-billionaires, I washed up at the staff level in the tax department of a financial services and insurance company in Boston. I'll call this company InsCo. I was shattered, ill, and downwardly mobile but was remarkably still able to land a professional job. With my Harvard degree, MBA, CPA, and my PwC experience, I felt like a damaged tropical bird blown into a litter-strewn inner city in a temperate climate. However much of a backward step this job might have seemed, I was thankful for it and did the best work I could in good faith. I was grateful to scrabble for crumbs with the dull-eyed and mite-ridden pigeons who were my new colleagues, and I ended up staying for fifteen years.

InsCo was large enough to be under continuous IRS audit, and a large part of my new job was tracking the information requests made by the IRS auditors. A group of us in the tax accounting department met with them weekly to review status, answer questions, and discuss next steps.

A side note: There are sections dealing with taxation and the insurance business in this book, including the following paragraph. For those readers not of the business world these sections may seem heavy, but they are fairly short. Please hang in there, as the payoffs are worth it.

There was a prominent category of information request that was not handled by me and was instead handled by the InsCo tax lawyers. These information requests related to LILOs (and their later cousins, the SILOs), pronounced "lie-lows," and standing for lease-in/lease-out. These were a complex scheme involving leases, interwoven legal structures, and large foreign infrastructure and transportation projects. Basically, they were prepackaged, promoted tax products that were sold to InsCo and other insurance companies by outside consultants with the promise of large upfront tax deductions and therefore tax savings. Then, decades later, the deductions would reverse, and the income tax would have to be paid. In the meantime, though, the insurance company would have the benefit of vast quantities of extra cash from delaying the payment of tax.

The LILOs didn't fool anyone involved in the audit. The real issue was that the enormous and deliberate complexity of the legal entity structures and agreements meant that the IRS, chronically understaffed and underfunded, had huge administrative burdens in pursuing tax justice. Over the four and a half years that I attended those meetings, as the tax lawyers alternately obfuscated over LILO facts, delayed delivering documents, and tried to negotiate with the IRS to retain some percentage of the LILO tax benefits, I came to understand that they were cynical schemes with no economic purpose other than tax evasion. InsCo was not actually a partner in the construction of a railroad yard in Austria or a hydroelectric dam in Canada, even though the LILO documents were designed to make it look like it was.

A few years after I joined the company, it was acquired by a financial services company (I'll call it ParCo) that had a larger global brand and presence. The moribund tax department where I worked was revitalized along with much of the company's finance sector. The top InsCo executives who had purchased and implemented the LILO product received huge stock and cash payouts when the company was acquired.

InsCo and the government were unable to agree on either compromise or settlement on the LILO issue during the audit. It took many years, but the LILOs went to tax court and the government prevailed. To my deep gratification, the tax benefits were ultimately completely disallowed.

My take on the LILOs is that InsCo paid some tens of millions of dollars to the consultants who were shilling them on the chance that InsCo would be able to negotiate a settlement with the IRS that would allow for some portion of the tax deductions in the early years. Even if the LILOs were completely disallowed, as they ended up being, InsCo had the cash up front and made a higher return on that cash than the IRS charged InsCo in interest. But the real payoff came from golden parachute executive compensation and severance arrangements upon the sale of the company to ParCo, InsCo having been made more attractive by the extra cash on its balance sheet.

During my time at InsCo, I learned that it received massive economic benefit from numerous tax schemes, not just the LILOs, and that many of the company's brightest minds were devoted to implementing and defending these various schemes. With taxes, there is what is called tax avoidance, meaning the right and even obligation every taxpayer has not to pay unnecessary taxes, and then there is tax evasion, meaning outright fraudulent or illegal tax positions. The problem with large companies like InsCo is that due to the complexity of their investments or the complexity of the business itself, there is an enormous gray area between avoidance and outright evasion.

But does it pass the sniff test, meaning does it basically stink? If the scheme obviously has no economic or business basis other than tax deferral or tax savings, then I call it tax exploitation, meaning it was cynically engineered by a black heart. Even if the dutiful small team of IRS auditors in your shop has to labor for fifteen years to bring the scheme to its knees, it is, in the end, a stinking turd.

In addition to reputation risk and pragmatic concerns such as disallowance of deductions and subsequent interest and penalty charges, there is a deeper price that companies pay when they opt for easy money from tax exploitation. The rot at the core of the company that is the cynical exploitation of tax loopholes and weak regulatory enforcement poisons the entire company from the top down. It is not possible for a company to devote massive energy to dissembling and at the same time achieve excellence in its core businesses and in managing its people. The leaders may present themselves as ethical, but the schizophrenia between the hidden urge to cheat and the outer shell of benevolence and auspicious intentions compromises their forward looking abilities.

# Chapter 25 - The Big Sick

~~~

Over the next several years at InsCo, I got promoted and also arranged for job transfers to acquire broader experience in the insurance and financial services industry. Once I had trouble with a cube neighbor deliberately banging file drawers closed when he learned that the loud noise bothered me, but I was lucky not to have dramatic flare-ups from any chemical exposures for the first ten years I was there.

Years seven through ten I spent at a small, highly profitable, and complex business unit I will call RINS. My time working on the IRS audit had sensitized me to cynical tax schemes. Unfortunately for me, around the time I joined RINS, management came up with a way to squeeze more profit out of the RINS cash cow by shifting a portion of its net income to an offshore affiliated legal entity. If they could work up a justification—and the complexity of this small business meant that once again convoluted agreements enabled false justifications—they could send about $8 million of taxable income every year to a ParCo company in Barbados. In this way, they could permanently save about $3 million of tax every year. I raised repeated and heated objections to the implementation of this agreement, arguing that it was unethical and had no business purpose other than tax evasion. The only result I achieved was damage to my long-term career prospects among my then colleagues. I was disappointed when the agreement was implemented and felt soiled by my proximity to it.

I became more disappointed at RINS as years passed and the quality of my work was not properly acknowledged. Also, the head of the business unit habitually made sexual innuendos and offensive gender-biased statements. I felt that his comments indicated chronic disregard and selfishness and that he no longer deserved the quality of my contributions to his group. I applied for a transfer that was also a promotion, and in mid-May of 2010 I started a new job in the long-term care (LTC) business unit within InsCo.

At this new job, I immediately developed serious debilitating symptoms. Near my cube was a room with about ten heavily used copy machines and printers. A vent from that room, by chance, had been misdirected and dumped near my cube. Probably these fumes were an initial trigger for my illness. The vent was corrected, but I still became acutely ill repeatedly. There was evidently a second contaminant, which was never identified but whose location I ultimately traced to an area of the floor that included my supervisor's office. This workspace contaminant was some spill or other residue that no one could smell and that was not detected by the standard workplace exposure tests for lead, volatile organic compounds, or airborne particulates.

This illness was tricky because the immediate indicators were slight brain fogginess and fatigue, which I was long accustomed to in my life and which I habitually ignored. The more dramatic symptoms did not appear for many hours after exposure. They got gradually worse during the twelve-hour period after the exposure, and they lasted for several days. Although my new job clearly caused my symptoms, at the beginning it was difficult to figure out which specific room, furniture, or other substance was making me ill.

Worst of all were the shocks inside my brain, like convulsions, sometimes with an accompanying buzzing or banging noise and occasionally with frightening hallucinations. I had these throughout the night, but they were worst as I was falling asleep. They were frequently triggered by noise, including tiny sounds like my pulse through my neck artery against the pillowcase or a little click inside my nasal passages or throat.

I had terrible trouble falling asleep and frequently woke up because of these shocks. Often, I only got one or two hours of sleep. I had temperature fluctuations and trouble regulating my body temperature with clothing and blankets. I also experienced unusual thirst, shooting pains in my arms and legs, achy skin, accelerated heartbeat, and extreme noise sensitivity. I had thoughts of despair and the feeling that everything was falling apart. The day after the exposure I suffered confusion, trouble recognizing common objects, more of the shocks, loss of physical coordination and dizziness, trouble with memory and language, irritability, fatigue, anxiety and the feeling that I was losing my reason, loss of physical stamina, and noise sensitivity. I also had trouble chewing and swallowing, and I bit the inside of my cheeks and my tongue frequently while eating.

If there wasn't a reexposure, subsequent days brought a gradual lessening of symptoms. I would have shocks without hallucinations, trouble falling asleep, long periods of wakefulness with negative thoughts, and most of the other symptoms of the first twenty-four hours, but not as bad. The total effect from a single primary exposure, meaning from the unidentified workspace contaminant, lasted up to five days. This manifestation was unlike anything I had ever experienced before.

At first, I did not make a connection between these acute symptoms and my lifelong ill health or even between these symptoms and the times I left college or left other jobs. The symptoms were so much worse and completely different, or at least I thought that at the time. I did not even recognize that all of the symptoms were neurological in nature. I thought if I tracked my movements at work daily, I could eventually figure out the source of the problem and avoid it in the future. In this way, I would be able to keep my job, which I was desperate to do after my history of career disruption. Through detailed and careful tracking of my symptoms and everywhere I went, after a couple of months I determined that the primary exposure was located in my supervisor's office. Even a short exposure of a few minutes in her office would trigger severe symptoms. As the months wore on, I became so ill and had such hopeless feelings and negative thoughts that I thought I was going to die.

While I was trying to figure it all out, I had no idea I was reopening an old wound within myself. In my ignorance of my own condition, I thought I could solve this problem as I had solved so many before in my life: through grit and determination and oblivious to my own suffering. This approach turned out to be tragically misguided.

These exposures and the terrible health effects didn't happen in a vacuum. I sought help from doctors, from my supervisors, and from people in the Human Resources department at work. I kept all sorts of people informed of my condition and struggles. I didn't receive support from any of these people. For many different reasons, no one stepped up to help me. I allowed the situation to continue for much longer than I should have because I didn't see with clarity the ultimate risk to my health for the rest of my life.

# Chapter 26 - The Worst Shock

Depression is not the right word for what I developed during that time at InsCo, when I was the most ill. It was beyond depression and more like mental anguish. It wasn't a gray fog of dullness, sadness, and self-disregard; it was instead dark thoughts about the future of the world and despair about my own fate. I imagined horrific scenarios where my sad flesh got a suppurating cancer, I had an accident, or Husband got ill or had an accident. My head was filled with images of flesh wounds, broken teeth, full-color tumors, and broken bones visible through torn flesh. These alternated with apocalyptic visions of societal and environmental devastation. This was not normal depression and was instead a waking nightmare state in which I was unable to escape the press of terrors.

During this time, I frequently thought about what I named "The Great Circle." This was a vision of human history in which people refused to bear the full costs of their consumption, which caused environmental destruction, which made people live with illness for long periods of their lives, which made them want to hoard assets against likely illness, which made them refuse to bear the full costs of their consumption, starting the circle around again. Wealth-owners deliberately spun the circle faster since toxic contamination is asset redistribution. This picture included a smaller and attached circle involving tax exploitation. Climate instability and global access to information are small beer next to the changes that chemicals are wreaking on humans, making them both addled and stupid. It seemed to me that these were the bleakest and also the most important truths and that I was the only one who knew them.

I don't mean to minimize the impact on others of standard depression (whatever that is), but there is a difference between dull sadness and continuous uncontrollable horrific visions of illness, destruction, and death. I told the doctors I saw at the time that I had dark thoughts, and not one asked me the nature of the thoughts. They didn't want to know and didn't have a healing framework for understanding and alleviating my anguish. On my side, I was too weak and devoid of words to be able to fully articulate it for them. From my lifelong struggles, I had become accustomed to sublimating my suffering. The few times I summoned the true grit to try to describe what I was feeling to these doctors, their disinterest made me feel inexplicably ashamed and as if I must be exaggerating my torment.

Now, years later, these horrific visions seem important, as though there are lessons to be learned about the true nature of some dementias and other varieties of mental illness. At these times cheerfulness and positive thoughts were not available to me because the chemistry of my brain had shifted. My mind was similar to that of Alzheimer's sufferers. These people can be crabby and even violent, incapable of affection or connection to others, and unable to see any good in the world. I wonder if they are tormented by horrific visions and unable to describe them, like I was. For rabies, it's the same thing. Surely the loss of uplifting and positive inclinations is equal to the deterioration of the self. To only manage horrifying and bleak thoughts is the same as to be dying.

It is cruel and ironic that chemical intolerance makes you tired, ill, and foggy, when you need stronger powers of charm, coherence, and stamina to convince your medical professionals that what you say makes sense. We are all more likely to connect with and believe people that we like, and doctors are no exception to this rule. My wan complexion, halting voice, and closed-down affect made me less likable, and these outward signs of my illness made it easier for them to dismiss my illness. I could have been an important case study, used by medical professionals to advance knowledge by illuminating the true effects of common chemicals on human health, but, instead, they tried to forget me as soon as they could.

One night after an exposure to the primary contaminant, meaning the area that included my supervisor's office, I had the worst of the shocks. The following is from my health log (unedited), dated August 23, 2010:

> *To sleep about eight fifteen. Sound shocks with body convulsions. High heartbeat (60 bpm). Very sleepy but unable to sleep. Thirsty, trouble regulating temperature. Thoughts of dismay. Semi-sat up for a while and drifted toward sleep. Then had a strange hallucination/shock. I felt like my skin and limbs were being blown away with a loud sound of wind and as if my chest was hollowed out and everything was dark and I couldn't breathe. I wanted to call for [Husband] but I couldn't. This feeling passed over me in three or four intensifying waves and then I forced myself out of it and awake. It felt like dying must feel like. Then I got up and turned on the light and felt fine—sleepy but OK. I remember worrying about my heart and feeling that [my*

*heart] was not OK. Awake for three hours by now. I ended up getting about two hours of sleep.*

I was not asleep, and this was not a dream. Instead, it was a neurological reality, by which I mean disruption so severe that a horrific alternative experiential reality was created. I now think that on that awful night, I did have an experience of neurological death but was somehow able to pull myself back from it.

Probably most people twitch a little sometimes when they are napping or when they are falling asleep. These are called sleep starts, and that is what my doctors told me I had. When I described my experience of these shocks to a neurologist, he wrote in my medical records (unedited):

> *The complaints the patient reports involve which [sic] she calls "shocks and convulsions" occurring at night, sometimes associated with a sound or with someone calling her name. The detailed descriptions of this are nothing more than normal sleep starts. She talks about some inability to sleep . . .*

This man demonstrated a criminal downplaying of my condition. The shocks I was having were way beyond sleep starts. They frequently were accompanied by a loud buzzing or banging sound, which is a characteristic of exploding head syndrome, in which a person hears noises that don't exist. When I got one of these shocks, I felt like someone had punched me inside my brain, and afterward I would lie awake for a while with my heart pounding and with dark thoughts—not the same as a muscle twitch.

The neurologist wrote, "The patient enters with a folder containing papers outlining all of her journals regarding her symptoms. She reads the experience of some of her symptoms out loud, and it sounds like she is reading a literary description from a novel." This was condescending and even unkind. He was anticipating review by colleagues and wanted to describe me in a way that diminished my credibility and justified his nonengagement with my condition. I had told him that I wrote things down because I didn't trust myself to remember them or describe them well because of the neurological damage. He was someone whose job it was to study impairments of the human brain, and loss of memory and language are key indicators of damage within his profession. He chose to portray my reliance on written notes in a way that diminished me and undermined my credibility, rather than admitting that it was an adaptation and a useful indicator of my condition.

Why were my doctors so completely hamstrung by my descriptions of my malady? It is obvious to me now that I was receiving repeated reinjuries to my nervous system, and yet they demonstrated a perverse and reality-denying bias against proper diagnosis. Partly they were angry with me for presenting them with a problem they couldn't solve. They each didn't want to be forced to defend their diagnosis, however commonsensical, against a workers' compensation tribunal. If they supported me, they would have been acting in defiance of the companies who actually footed the bill for health insurance, long-term disability insurance, and workers' compensation insurance. These companies indirectly paid their salaries. They looked at me and saw trouble for themselves. Nothing in their administrative support structure or professional culture encouraged them to align themselves with me. These early doctors, who could have saved me from permanent disability, were instead motivated by desperation to evade engagement with a widely discredited and politically unpopular condition, namely chemical intolerance, also called multiple chemical sensitivities.

I had told the neurologist several times that I couldn't actively smell the toxin and that the symptoms appeared many hours after exposure. Yet his primary suggestion to me at the end of our consultation was that my condition could be managed through psychological conditioning. He said I could be trained to control the physical manifestations of my responses to smells I encountered through a cognitive feedback mechanism. How was I supposed to control my bodily reactions when I couldn't smell the trigger? At a time when I was having these shocks (like seizures), which were frequent during the day and continuous at night, and I was having trouble recognizing common objects, finding words, and chewing and swallowing, he ordered *no* neurological testing. Instead, he wrote in his summary, "The impression is that clinically I suspect nothing neurologically of any significance."

It is common sense that the human body can be injured by a toxic substance such that some basic functions and balances are impaired and later easily reinjured. Given my medical and life history, suggesting the illness had a psychological basis and that my physical symptoms could somehow be alleviated by the exercise of willpower was equivalent to saying that I had the power to control the illness. This suggests it was my own fault if I didn't stop the symptoms from occurring, which is outrageous. Shame on these doctors and the medical profession in general for not helping me and for acting from self-protecting and insular motivations instead of empathic curiosity and the true desire to heal.

We need a new medical science that deals with the effect of chemicals on our neurological and adrenal systems. Our current medical system is not adequate, and the pressures of the capitalist faith have, so far, obstructed the acquisition of true knowledge in this area. Large companies are motivated by profits and heedlessly release toxic products into the marketplace. We are entering a new era in which the explosion of untested chemicals in our everyday lives means that conditions like mine are in turn destined to explode in frequency. People like me cannot be marginalized forever. If doctors and workers' compensation boards deny realities in front of them because the current diagnosis guidelines are not sufficient, new guidelines must be developed.

We need devices that can detect, identify, and measure potentially as well as proven toxic chemicals in our homes, our cars, and the wider world. We also need devices and testing approaches that can detect, identify, and measure the impairments suffered by humans. Surely there are indicators in the blood or other easily tested bodily components that could assist in detecting and measuring the sort of disruption I suffer. We are tender lumps of flesh and bone, susceptible to easy damage. To imagine that we exist outside of the rules of everyday commonsense science and are immune to the toxic soup around us is dangerous fantasy.

I think I died the night of my worst shock, when my skin, flesh, and bones were blown away in a gray swirling wind. Instead of lungs and entrails, there was a yawning tattered cavity below my partial shoulders, with frayed pinkish bits of my spine and ribs at the back. I gasped for air and the power to call out. I was weighed down and yet floating in a soft and empty dark space, my mind desperate for the comfort of my loved one, whose name I couldn't form. Probably infants left in hot cars have similar visions of neurological horror before they die from the superheated noxious chemicals around them. It is likely that as a small child, before and after I was in the coma from that first chemical exposure, I had the same horrific visions. Even though I was preverbal and didn't have words to describe them, these experiences wore dark pathways in my brain. I sometimes blame myself for accepting the way my family treated me, but perhaps it was these ancient trails of sadness and loss that made me the way I am. It was these submerged memories of violent trauma that made me susceptible to hopes of kindness and likely to overlook indications of secret disregard in the people I loved and from whom I wanted love.

# Chapter 27 - How Many Beans Make Five

∽

In 2010 when I became so ill, I kept my supervisor, Caroline, and also folks in Human Resources (HR) informed of the progress of my illness. At first I thought I was the only one with symptoms, but after I was there a few months, Caroline called my attention to the many young women with unusual hair loss in the business unit. She herself had unexplained anxiety, depressive thoughts, thinning hair, and an unusual bald spot on her head, all of which she associated with her workspace. The female head of the business unit had also complained to Caroline about her own thinning hair, and this woman had associated her hair loss with "the carpets." I wrote an email query to the previous occupant of Caroline's office, someone considerably above my station whom I knew casually, and this woman said that she struggled with environmental sensitivities currently and also had when she worked in that office space. The very day that I became convinced that it was Caroline's office that was making me ill and told her so, she made arrangements to move out of it herself.

I brought these cases to the attention of my HR contact but ultimately felt that the company wasn't adequately acknowledging the health risks of the workplace to its employees. But it was a subtler impact that should have gotten the attention of the folks in charge, if only for pragmatic reasons. This is the story.

When I joined the LTC business unit in 2010, it was a time of turmoil in the industry and a time of crisis in my new business unit. The company was losing a lot of money on the long-term care insurance policies that it had sold in the past. Each new policy it sold would likely lose money as well. The problem was that over the prior fifteen years or so, certain assumptions had been made as part of key calculations for the premiums that were charged. These assumptions ended up being so wrong that ultimately the business was not viable because premiums were way, way too low. The magnitude of the past mistakes relating to premium pricing was impressive—a $3.2 billion loss per the company's September 2010 reporting. The company had a contractual obligation to maintain the policies it had already provided to customers for as long as these customers wanted them, and it was not allowed to increase prices without the approval of state regulators. Future premiums needed to increase by a whopping 40 percent for about 80 percent of their customers for the business to be viable in the future and also to offset the pricing mistakes of the past. If the company was able to get these ambitious price increases past the regulators, they projected they could make up about $2.2 billion of the $3.2 billion. So, optimistically assuming that the future price increases were sufficient and would be approved, InsCo estimated that the net loss reflecting the trouble the business was in was just over a billion dollars.

The company didn't want to sell any new policies given the risk of losing yet more money, but state regulators were less likely to approve premium price increases if the company didn't plan to stay in the market. The company was in a bind. They wanted the $2.2 billion in their pocket that would come from future price increases, but they didn't want to be in the LTC business anymore.

The solution was to tell everyone, meaning customers, the public, industry analysts, state regulators, and all staff below top leadership, that they intended to keep offering new LTC policies for the indefinite future. This way the state regulators would approve the large price increases on existing policies. Then, as soon as all of the requested price increases were approved, the company would stop selling new policies, basically exiting the market in contradiction to everything they previously said they planned to do. (I am conjecturing all of this. No one ever told me this was InsCo's strategy, but I intuited it at the time.) And in September of 2016, a short time after InsCo's LTC business unit pushed all of their price increases through the state regulators, they did exit the market!

It was demanding for senior leadership to pursue this hidden devious strategy while projecting fake sincerity and fake good faith in the day-to-day running of the business. The company had transferred a few tough-minded superstars into the LTC business unit to manage this tricky transition. As I look back on the responses of my supervisors to my illness, I can see that these people had an enormous hidden agenda on their minds at that time. The gnawing secret that top leadership shared partially explains the extreme lack of empathy I encountered as I became more and more ill. The people who ran the business, with whom I worked daily, did not want to hear that I suspected an odorless horror was emanating from their workspaces. They wanted good news and healthy compliant staff as they made plans to gut the business, not distractions such as possible environmental remediation or me looking distinctly ill and wearing a half-face respirator. My supervisor's supervisor started asking me when I planned to leave. From the way he and others treated me, I felt like someone in a nineteenth-century factory who was fired for losing an arm in badly maintained machinery.

Probably the most important technical calculations that this business unit had performed in past years were the calculations of premium prices. Similarly, the most important technical calculations it would be performing in the coming years would be the calculations of the increased premium prices it wanted to charge in the future to send along with supporting packages to the regulators for approval. The people who were to execute these calculations, who are called pricing actuaries, were in offices next to Caroline's and had been there for years. These two mature men didn't look well. One of them had stacks of files a few feet high everywhere in his office, indicating either eccentricity or a disorder, and both of them had bad skin color and a constant worried look on their faces. Their affects were similar in this regard and were the same as that of a third long-term staff member who was in a cube on the other side of Caroline's office. All three men looked slightly anxious and unwell all of the time.

Actuaries tend to be the smartest people around, and they are the people with the deepest understanding of any insurance business. Yet, within this failing business, the actuaries, whom the company should have been able to rely on to provide the motive force to make the best of a bad situation, were being poisoned by their offices. I could see it on their faces. How long had they been ill? Was the unidentified spilled toxin the indirect reason for the pricing mistakes of the past? Whatever their considerable gifts, were these impaired people likely to generate the absolute best answers and strategies for this troubled business unit at a time of such industry turmoil and with such high stakes?

Just as people who are ill are unable to do their best work, people who are lying are unable to make the best decisions. If leadership in that business unit had not been distracted by the lies they were telling outsiders about their future intentions and instead had had the mental space and open minds to listen to what I was telling them about something nasty in the workspace, they would have been able to anticipate the potential adverse effects on these men whom they needed to be at the absolute top of their game—not to mention the adverse effects on all of the supporting staff members, and even themselves.

I can't pretend that I am anywhere near as smart as the people who were running that business at that time. But what use was all that intelligence if their impaired perceptions made them unable to recognize and act on such a threat right in front of them? Once I was in a meeting with these people, and I felt so ill I had to put my head down on the conference table in front of me. At that point I had moved to an empty work area on a different floor of the building, and sometimes I worked from home. I walked around wearing a respirator. I sent regular email updates on my condition and progress. I looked terrible. I was providing these business leaders almost daily with evidence of the toxins in their space. This evidence was reality-based information that could have helped them and their staff make better decisions in the future. However, because their minds were full of willful and exploitative deception, they were not able to connect with the gift of knowledge I was offering.

# Chapter 28 - The Wall of Books

A few months after I moved into the LTC office space and suffered repeated exposures to the unidentified primary toxin in Caroline's office, I developed a secondary intolerance to a broad range of common chemicals. This is the intolerance that I still have. These secondary exposures triggered the same range of symptoms, but they were not as bad as from the primary toxin. My nervous system had become so damaged through repeated reinjuries by the primary toxin that even tiny amounts of secondary exposure would cause debilitating illness. I continued my careful note-taking of exposures and symptoms. The range of substances I was sensitive to quickly broadened to include fragrances, smells, and chemicals used in just about every office, restaurant, public building, mode of transport, and medical facility, and most people's homes. I became intolerant of many food additives and most ingredients in personal care products. My reaction was not allergic or allergen based. Instead, it was based on an acquired intolerance or sensitivity from my repeated chemical injuries.

After struggling for almost a year at the LTC job, I left the company. Although no one in the medical profession had helped me to understand my condition, I finally and fully understood that I had suffered terrible damage to my long-term health by staying in that workspace as long as I did. I was ill and demoralized. I hadn't received support from anyone at work or any doctors I had seen to receive long-term disability or workers' compensation benefits, so I knew I still needed to work and earn money.

My replacement at my previous job at the small RINS business unit of InsCo had struggled, and there had been many mistakes since my departure. I sent my prior boss at RINS a chatty email to let him know I had left the company and why. He, able to read between the lines, wrote back and offered me a job. Within a month of leaving the company, I'd been hired back at my previous position and workspace at RINS. This was mid-2011, a year after I had transferred away from that job because I didn't feel appreciated and because the head of RINS regularly said sexual and other objectionable things about women. Now I'd returned, once again grateful to have a job given my compromised health and my lack of professional success in the meantime.

The folks from this earlier job knew me well and were sympathetic to my condition. Initially I worked mostly from home. Then the toilets at work were renovated and I couldn't find one without fragranced air fresheners, so I worked exclusively from home in an informal disability accommodation. I was comfortable with the work itself and brought my A game to get the group back in shape and correct the disorder that had accumulated during my absence.

I struggled to recover from the terrible traumas I had suffered during the previous year. I also struggled to manage new adverse exposures and episodes of illness. I kept meticulous notes to learn all of the things that made me ill, but it was still difficult to identify the specific exposures because the symptoms were delayed. Also, the effects sometimes lasted a few days, so the exposures became cumulative and layered. Often it was nearly impossible to figure out what exactly had caused the adverse response, which doomed me to repeated painful episodes until I finally identified the culprit. A typical entry contains my suspicions about processing residues or other toxic aspects of newly purchased clothing:

> *Lay awake for a while and then light sleep. Same pattern as when I handled new clothes before, and in fact I did handle new clothes. Large load of pink pajama trousers into the wash machine and then out. Surprised since they had been washed and then aired out, but I find that just a little exposure to that stuff has a large effect on me. No shocks, just disrupted/light sleep.*

A week later I surmised the exact component that was causing me trouble:

> *Occasional trouble from the new clothes—why do I keep fooling with them?! This time I'm pretty sure it was the toxic-smelling waistband in the new flannel trousers. Must throw them all away (bite the bullet)!*

By the time I returned with my tail between my legs to the job I had been so pleased to be rid of a year before, my interests and passions outside of work had vanished. Entire bodies of knowledge, memory, and concern had fallen away. The focus of my life had become to get by and survive, hopefully while not in a depressed and fatigued state with banging noises inside my head. Before I became ill, I had developed an interest in making small-scale sculptures, like shadow boxes. This interest was an evolution of my lifelong passions for handwork and collecting small material-culture treasures like tools, sewing notions, snapshots, and ephemera. When I became ill, this activity stopped. My life became smaller and more constricted as I slowly grew to accept that I could not do normal things. Over the next few years, as I built a bare-bones life using unconventional approaches to many of the activities of daily living, I was able to claw back more days of wellness than illness. With the intermittent wellness came a new clarity of mind about my life history and my current situation. As I continued to be made ill by everyday objects and substances, I began to see these objects and substances clearly.

It is not necessary to have in your apartment or house the traditional middle-class wall of books. Most of these books are printed with toxic inks, and the paper and glues also have chemicals in them. It would be better for your health and that of your family if you didn't have walls of books inside your living space. Here is a test: take a recently published picture book, close your eyes, open the book to a random spot, and place your nose next to the open page. Inhale slowly and deeply. Consider: Would you want to take a nap with your face on this surface? Would you want your infant child or grandchild to take a nap with his or her face on this surface? Or, does a little voice tell you this could harm the child? Leave aside any assumption you might have that it is safe; concentrate on the smell, and trust your instincts.

Perhaps your sense of smell doesn't raise alarms with a picture book. Try it with a magazine. Then consider that you may not want piles of magazines inside the space where you and your family live. One would think that a *National Geographic* magazine is all good, but if you view it with absolute clarity, you will recognize that it is a terrible smelling and even dangerous object.

Books and magazines are only one example. Try to see clearly the other objects inside your home. What are they made of? How about packaging, which might sit in the house for a while after you bring new purchases home? Probably you have already realized that most junk mail has a vile smell. Then there are the materials that went into the construction of your home itself. Think clearly about what these materials are made of. Do you want your new infant child or grandchild breathing in the smells coming from these materials? Consider any fragranced products you have in your home. Maybe they smell nice, but consider that the smell you find attractive could be masking a second smell that would otherwise alert you to its toxic nature. These substances affect me strongly, but they are harmful at some level to everyone. Even if people can't consciously sense them, no one is immune to their toxic nature. From my own experience, I know truths that our society has not yet developed the testing equipment to "scientifically" confirm. We are being lied to about the safety of the chemicals in the products that surround us.

# Chapter 29 - The Bedbug

Although the breach with my parents when I was in my late twenties turned out to be final, I maintained contact with my siblings and my mother's two sisters. Considering our similar personal attributes and interests, it made sense for me and my mother's older sister, Cynthia, to be friends. We were both cheerful, easygoing, childless people who knew a lot about art and liked to eat. In 2012, she was in her late seventies and I was fifty. She lived happily in a small co-op in the Upper East Side of New York City, and I was only a four-hour train ride away in the Boston area. After a long and distinguished career as a research psychologist and teacher of psychology, she was orchestrating a staggered retirement from a high-level administrative position in the psychology department of a prominent New York City university. She continued to provide dissertation guidance to a handful of graduate students, traveled frequently to less-popular Asian destinations on tours that emphasized cultural history, gave docent tours at the Asia Society, and volunteered at the Metropolitan Museum of Art. She was a tall, slender, highly educated woman with a charismatic, self-assured presence. She had been unapologetically well-dressed and beautiful her whole life.

Cynthia imagined herself basking in the success of brokering a reconciliation between my mother and me, so she started to cultivate a friendship with me and Husband. I wanted to have family members in my life. In case I was mentioned in this wealthy relative's will, I wanted our friendship to justify any such bequest. Not that an inheritance from Cynthia was imminent, as her own health and mobility were those of someone twenty-five years younger, her mother lived to her nineties after smoking heavily for at least sixty years, and her mother's mother was well over a hundred when she died.

In the spring of 2012, Cynthia came for a visit of a few days, during which time Husband cooked many lovely meals and she and I went out and about in Boston. I was careful and lucky with exposures, so was in good spirits. I told her in broad strokes about how I had to quit my job at InsCo in the LTC business unit, how I had clawed my way back to employment, and how ill I had been. I told her I carefully tracked exposures and their effects on my health. She was also aware that Husband struggled with chemical intolerance and that both of our lives were somewhat fraught with long-term illness.

Several months later she came for another visit, which at first proceeded much as the first one, with many pleasant meals and outings to museums. Then one evening as we sat together in the living room, she mentioned a spider in her apartment that was biting her every night. She showed me little red bumps on her upper arm, side torso, and neck, and said what a relief it was to get away from "that damn spider" for a few days. I said to her calmly, "Those look like bedbug bites. You'll probably want to look into that when you get back." And indeed, the marks had the classic "breakfast, lunch, dinner" pattern of three bites close together that bedbugs give. There had recently been press about the explosion of bedbugs in New York's Upper East Side and how appalled the high-toned residents were by their stigma. Bedbugs are notorious for hitching rides on luggage, but since she had already been in our house for a few days, there wasn't anything useful Husband and I could do or say to prevent infestation. She stayed for the rest of the visit as planned.

Our house was a reasonably safe haven from the outside world, which for us was full of invisible toxins. We were used to being made ill in our everyday activities, but the prospect of bedbug remediation, which would naturally include insecticides, was unimaginable. I started to have nightmares about bedbugs and spent anxious waking hours imagining the different routes by which they would make their way through our house. By chance, I got some actual spider bites one night, which caused me even more anxiety.

A few weeks after her visit, Cynthia called in some agitation. She had hired a pest control expert, and she did have bedbugs, she admitted. She apologized repeatedly for visiting when they existed inside her apartment. I quizzed her about her suitcase-packing protocol relative to her bed and about other details of her infestation. It turned out that all her immediate neighbors had had bedbugs, she had known about many of these occurrences before coming to visit, and it was understood within her apartment building that there were critter conduits like floorboard cracks between the apartments. The expert had advised her to pack all her loose belongings into airtight plastic bins for the six months required for the bedbugs to die, and in the meantime her apartment would be sprayed and all cracks sealed with foams and caulk. She offered to pay for spraying if it turned out our house had become infested. The problem was that Husband and I could not tolerate spraying like normal people could. Exposure to insecticide would make us ill—probably for a long time, since the adverse effects of the insecticide would linger. Possibly we would be forced to sell our house and move.

With this confirmation, financial and general life devastation loomed large, partly because our long-term illnesses affected our levels of mental resilience. What level of magical thinking and denial had to have been going on for Cynthia to be bitten *every night* before the visit, get the three-bite pattern all over her arms and torso, hear from her neighbors at the regular co-op meetings and in passing about their problems with bedbugs, and yet tell herself that visiting me, who had been terribly ill and still struggled daily with chemical intolerance, was a good idea? Husband and I started calling her "The Bedbug."

My mother's younger sister, Gloria, is a social worker and therapist. Gloria and I wrote and chatted a few times a year generally, and she called me shortly after Cynthia told me the bedbug news. Cynthia had visited her in Denver a couple of months before she came to see me, and Gloria and her husband noticed a dead bedbug in Cynthia's effects. They immediately contacted local pest control companies and researched extermination approaches for their type of house in their region. They knew Cynthia was planning to visit me but *didn't alert me.* They also didn't firmly tell Cynthia not to travel further until she resolved the problem.

Before she visited Gloria, Cynthia had visited my mother, Polly, in Hometown and stayed with my younger sister, Amy. Gloria said to me, "As I said to Polly, thank God she didn't give Amy bedbugs—can you imagine how awful that would have been for her, with the children?" What were these women not hearing about my illness and struggles? How could Gloria and my mother discuss the possible effects of bedbugs on Amy, knowing that Cynthia's visit to me was in the works yet not preventing that visit? Had it registered with them that I was seriously ill, or were all three so oblivious as to be delusional?

Sometimes it takes me a while to fully accept that a given relationship is a stinker. Although I didn't talk to Cynthia with the same frankness and enthusiasm as before, I did chat with her on the phone a few times over the next year or so. For the last of these, she called me, as she had for the others. She had an assessing and distant tone, as though she had come to a conclusion and had a strategic agenda. After a little chitchat, she asked me three questions in quick succession: How many of those box sculptures have you made, anyway? Has Husband sold any of his photographs recently? What does Husband do with himself all day? Both of us had been ill for a long time. We struggled to address those exact issues in our lives. She already knew the sad answers and was only going through the motions of asking the questions to establish that she had given me a chance to justify myself.

Cynthia had failed to broker a reconciliation between Mom and me. Worse, she had failed to understand how ill I was and had been careless. She needed to rewrite the story so that instead of my breaking up with her, she was breaking up with us because we were losers. Asking those questions was only a performance with the hidden purpose to judge us wanting. Big thing for Cynthia: offload the losers. Not much nuance there. After this telephone call, I was done with Cynthia, and she was done with me.

∞

The best bedbug prevention and probably also remediation is to maintain a mixed-species population of spiders in your house. Naturally this solution is not suggested by experts in the pest control industry, but it is the job of spiders to eat bedbugs. Maybe it was our own spiders that saved us from Cynthia's bedbugs, or maybe it was luck. These days I'm careful to vacuum around these tiny and patient sentinels or gently transport them outside, instead of sucking them up.

# Chapter 30 - Call with Kirsten

Around the time I returned to the RINS business unit, I remembered I had been in an unexplained coma when I was an infant. I made the connection between my adult neurological impairment and this childhood event. At first, any suggestion of causal linkage seemed outlandish, but the more I thought about the similarities, the more convinced I became. I saw that I had been quiet and reserved as a small child for the same reasons I had trouble finding words in job workspaces that made me ill, namely loss of language due to neurological injury. I understood for the first time that I had been withdrawn and depressed for periods of time as a child. The extreme mental distress I suffered from ongoing chemical exposures was an echo of my childhood depression.

It was common sense to me that a human organism could receive a neurological injury from exposure to a toxic chemical that then made that organism less resilient to other chemicals and environmental toxins in the future. But the doctors I had seen were unhelpful and sometimes hurtful. Perhaps because they were so awful, it was easier to reject their conclusions completely and adopt a maverick approach to solving the mystery. Over the next couple of years, I gnawed on this bone, worrying it and trying to remember episodes of illness, depression, or inexplicable behavior from the distant past, along with details of my workspaces or living spaces during each episode. I began to wonder if my parents knew what had happened and hid it from me. Then in 2013, after our father died, I got a call from my older sister, Kirsten.

With true grit, Kirsten had reinvented herself after leaving Hometown for college, casting off her fat and becoming slender and extremely athletic. She was pretty, with soft and naturally fragrant skin and low-maintenance yet flattering haircuts that framed her enormous eyes. I never learned how to buy suitable clothing and felt poor and unworthy in Patagonia-type retail stores, but she had no such doubts. She dressed well and with ease. Also unlike me, she made and retained close female friends and had a working bullshit meter.

Our relationship improved after high school but remained lopsided. She never wanted to be with me as much as I wanted to be with her, and her treatment of me reflected this inequality. As an example, during my time off from college when I was nineteen and living in Hometown, she came home from college for Christmas. My parents had not invited me to the family festivities only a couple of blocks from my apartment, but Kirsten made a big fuss about how the two of us would get together afterward. She went out with friends instead and came by hours later and with a friend in tow. She and her friend didn't sit down. Instead, Kirsten demanded that I lend her my diaphragm since she hadn't packed hers for her trip home. I refused for about five silent reasons, among them that I doubted she would clean it properly, if that were even possible, and she left in a huff. Every time I remember this incident, the vision of an invisibly damaged female prophylactic device flashes through my brain and I realize I would have never trusted it subsequently if I had lent it to her.

Kirsten had stayed in Boulder, Colorado, after attending law school there. I have only a few letters from her from the almost forty years since we lived in the apartment by ourselves. One, a postcard, begins, "Thank you for your recent letter and for the ones before that." The man she married had grown up not far from Boston, and for many years I intuited that they came through town regularly to visit his family but did not get in touch with me, which hurt my feelings. When she did make arrangements to visit, Husband and I were often inconvenienced by delays or last-minute cancellations. Then there was an acute rancorous episode that was probably orchestrated by our younger sister, and afterward we weren't in touch for five or six years until after Dad died.

It was natural for us to check in given his recent death. Kirsten had made one child, was divorced, was bitter toward her ex-husband, and seemed neurotic and unhappy. According to the terms of Dad's will, each of his three daughters was to receive 1 percent of the value of his estate, with the remaining 97 percent going to Hunter. Kirsten wanted to know if I was poor, so she said in a fake-concerned tone, "I suppose it must be very hard for you to receive so little money from Dad, especially if you need the money." I responded evasively and was on alert—this badly disguised schadenfreude was more typical of our teenage years and suggested a renewed congealing of ill will.

However, there was a chance Kirsten could shed some light on my health history, and, in good faith, I wanted to inform her of what was important in my life. After we each managed to convey to the other that we were reconciled to Dad's bequests and hadn't expected anything fair or conciliatory from him, I told her about my planned move out of the Boston area and that it was necessary because of my illness. She expressed no curiosity or sympathy about the details of my ill health or my career disruptions. Instead, she said that others in the family were also sensitive to coffee or certain foods. *Not quite the same thing*, I thought, but I didn't argue with her.

I mentioned a possible connection between my lifelong symptoms of ill health, my chemical intolerance, and my illness as a baby. I said I suspected my childhood neurological collapse was due to a chemical exposure of some kind. Immediately, I had her pinpoint attention. She spoke quickly and said only the following words: "Do you know how it happened?" I was taken aback by the directness of her words and the urgency in her voice. I said I didn't and how could I? The mood of the call then shifted completely, and she became much quieter, as though her mind was spinning. By then she had been a lawyer for almost thirty years, and I sensed she was calling on her professional experience to know when to shut the fuck up. She indicated she was done with the call. I told her I would email her some pictures of our planned house purchase, which I did, and she said she would send me her new home address and phone number via email, which she didn't.

I'm slow on the uptake; I know this. I know I deny unpleasant realities about family members or friends to preserve relationships. I know the truth stares me in the face and I look away because I must accommodate someone's weakness or even ill intent to keep that person in my life. But this time, from her tone of voice when she asked me if I knew how it had happened, I finally picked up on the messages from Kirsten. I completely understood that Mom had confided to Kirsten the circumstances of my childhood chemical exposure, at least in broad strokes. Meaning, I was right, and it *had* happened.

My powers of cross-examination are pitiable, but were they supernatural my sister would not have told me all she knew, so I forgive myself for not questioning her further during that phone call. She had never respected my own need for information and was long accustomed to viewing me as a reject from the sorority between herself and our mother. Despite my suffering, she didn't feel any obligation to give me even crucial information that could have helped me manage my life-altering illness because that information might have compromised our mother.

It took me a while to articulate all that I had learned. Odd, how an idea stays amorphous until the proper words are attached to it. Husband had always thought that the relationship between my older sister and me was not a healthy one, and I agree with him now. But it is still hard to accept that she knew important things about me and didn't tell me. If Kirsten had cared, she would have understood that the doctors I consulted would have been forced to take my condition more seriously if I knew for sure it was from a childhood exposure. This would have changed how I managed the illness because I would have no longer been alone. The doctors would have been forced to step up concerning other support I needed but wasn't getting, like long-term disability benefits or workers' compensation. My sister didn't care about any of this.

What else does she know? Probably many other secrets about family members. Through these inappropriate adult confidences, Mom created a divide, with the two of them on one side and the subjects of the secrets on the other. Kirsten grew to believe that she was not obligated to treat people with empathy. She became accustomed to deriving personal power from judging others and behaving selfishly, and, as a grown woman, she was unable to be cheerful, truly supportive, and loving toward the poor bastard she married.

After chewing on this phone call for a while, I realized Mom's approach when discussing me with other family members was to minimize both the weight of my illness and also my worth generally. When Kirsten reminded me that I wasn't the only one sensitive to coffee, she was recycling conversations between herself and Mom in which they downplayed what had happened to me. This way Mom could sort of admit aspects of the truth while making light of my experiences and my value. When these other family members then talked to me, they would get the impression that I was exaggerating my struggles, which then caused further distance between them and me. I see now that when Gloria and the Bedbug observed me, although their expressions appeared to be open and friendly, their faces were actually veiled. My aunts were so busy filtering their impressions through Mom's interpretations that they were unable to experience true concern and connection.

When I was so ill and preparing to leave my job in 2011, my aunts knew I was a primary breadwinner yet they did not offer to help me financially. They knew my parents wouldn't. I had supposedly affectionate relationships with these two mature and prosperous women. I was likely too proud to accept money from them, but I would have been encouraged by the gesture if they had offered. This absence of assistance wasn't reasonable given my life circumstances. Instead, during one phone call with Gloria, I became tearful when talking about my long history of bad sleep and how demoralizing it was to feel ill so often. "I just feel so damaged," I said, despairing, and Gloria answered with a firm denial. "Nonsense, there is nothing the matter with you. You are a lovely young woman." Gloria's words of supposed comfort made me feel deeply discouraged and alienated. In her willful ignorance, she wasn't capable of reconciling my reality with her world view, which in this case was actually Mom's world view. Once again the circumstances around my illness exposed the weakness in a relationship with someone whom I had wrongly believed to be a true friend. She didn't intend to hurt me, but I had some trouble bouncing back after this fresh evidence of how unlucky I had been, in health and in birth family. To keep me grounded in my own truth and at the risk of unkindness toward Gloria, I turned one of Husband's humorous mottos into a new and brutalist credo: "Beware the stupid people, for they will fuck you up."

It seems cheesy to follow the money, but largesse is an indicator of consideration. From my maternal grandmother's estate, loaded up with tracts of ancestral Kansas farmland and groaning with blue chip portfolios, I received $4,000 via Mom. I now see clearly that what Gloria and the Bedbug sent me over the years was occasional, meager, and sometimes depressing shipments of vintage junk. I always felt disappointed, not because I'm greedy or ungrateful, but because I discerned the underlying gift of thin affection. In the future, I will only accept friendship from big hearts—Elizabeth Warren, Roxane Gay, Jennifer Saunders, Amy Goodman. If any of these ladies come knocking on my door, I will answer it and step outside. If not, I will just stay home.

# Chapter 31 - Medical Case History

As I tracked the exposures that made me ill, I was forced to acknowledge there were problems with the Boston-area two-family house we lived in at the time that could not be corrected. Our neighbors' houses were close on either side, and, by bad luck, both of their laundry vents pointed toward us. Both neighbors also replaced their driveway surfaces and used a highly toxic asphalt sealant that, for a few years, made a terrible smell in the summertime. Between the fragranced dryer sheets and the truly ghastly asphalt sealant, I couldn't spend time in the yard or even open a window without taking a chance of being ill for a few days. We also had tenants who, despite our emphatic guidance, used products that left residual fragrances in our rental unit. I couldn't enter that space unless I was wearing a respirator mask, and we had to tape over the cracks around the door in our apartment that led to the shared front hall to prevent these smells from oozing into our space.

There was no question of moving locally—the Boston real estate market was loaded up with overpriced junk. Because we needed to have space around the house, meaning expensive suburbs, there wasn't anything in our price range that would have been safe for me. In 2013, we put our own overpriced piece of junk on the market, we chose a new home in Western Massachusetts very, very carefully, I told folks at my job that my phone number had changed, and we got the fuck out of Dodge.

I have been able to build a healthier life in our small town in Franklin County. Our home renovation used only nontoxic materials and we are far enough away from neighbors' laundry vents that the house is safe for me. Gradually my baseline health has improved. However, to avoid adverse exposures, my movements and life actions are extremely limited. I carry a cartridge-filter half-face respirator with me when I go anywhere out of the house, but even it is not completely effective for all potential exposures.

I am unable to travel or ride on public transport. Most cars make me ill. For a while, we owned a thirty-year-old car because newer cars have a plastic smell. That old car, though, had fluid leaks that made me ill, and when it was repaired the engine burned off spills that also made me ill. We got rid of it, and now we have no car. Some car companies such as Ford and Volvo have cleaned up their car interior components, but not enough for me to be able to ride in them without a mask. If I am riding in a friend's car, which I occasionally do, I wear my respirator and have the windows open as much as possible.

My diet is restricted. When I go to a restaurant, I usually become ill because of fragrances or cleaning products, so I almost never go out to eat. I become ill from the lobby of my bank unless the visit is brief and I am wearing my respirator. For a while, I was able to go to the YMCA because they had a no-fragrance policy. Then they changed their cleaning-product suite, and I was made ill for a few months before I figured it out and quit the Y. I don't go to the movies, the mall, shops, museums, or concerts.

Most recently published books make me ill, as do newspapers and magazines. I can't go to the library without my mask, and even then I keep the visit short. I have to be careful with printed materials and mail delivered to my home. I need to be careful with any new consumer product that we bring into the house, such as clothing, electronics, or tools. The mold-release compounds on many molded plastic components make me ill. So do many items made of rubber because of chemicals added to most rubbers during manufacture. I can't use normal soap. I can't use dry cleaning. I avoid standing next to most people unless it is breezy outside because of their laundry fragrances or body care fragrances. We tell friends not to use fragrance or fragranced laundry products if they come over, but this is not always successful.

In an office environment, whiteboard markers, magic markers, color printouts, tape, packing tape, adhesive surfaces, some pens, cardboard boxes, cleaning products, and especially toilet air fresheners all make me ill, along with furniture, carpets, and cushions containing formaldehyde, foams, and glues.

If I do have an exposure, the symptoms are so debilitating that it isn't tolerable. It would not be possible for me to go to a job or into an environment where I am exposed to these things. It isn't just that I am tired; it is instead that my sleep is quite disrupted with exploding head shocks, I lie awake for a long time with dark thoughts, and I feel malaise and fatigue the next day. I bite the inside of my mouth and have trouble chewing and swallowing. I have trouble finding words, concentrating, and remembering. I'm unable to interact normally with people, and I have a tendency to say inappropriate things that might be hurtful to people when I don't intend to hurt anyone. I also repeat myself and speak in ways that don't make sense in the immediate context. If I'm ill, the fatigue keeps me from doing things that I need to do, like take a bath or clean the house.

I want to help others who might have similar conditions, so in the spirit of medical case histories and in the interest of completeness, here are more medical details.

When I was the most ill in 2010 and 2011, I was about forty-nine years old. I started to have perimenopausal symptoms. My menstrual cycle became irregular, and I skipped periods. My breasts became enormous, bloated, sore things with frequent stabbing pains. I had mid-cycle blood spotting and hot flashes. My libido, ever a tender flower, basically disappeared, and I had vaginal dryness and weight gain. When my baseline health started to improve in 2013 and 2014, all of these symptoms disappeared. My breasts shrank to their normal size, my periods became regular again, and I lost the weight I had gained. My earlier extreme neurological and adrenal distress absolutely triggered the hormonal changes that caused these temporary perimenopausal symptoms. The connection between chemical injury, neurological imbalance, and hormonal difficulty must have been the cause of my menstrual pain and chronic premenstrual distress even before my illness at age forty-eight. This means that my childhood chemical injury messed up my hormones along with the neurological adverse effects.

I always had thin hair compared to my mother and sisters, and, when I was the most ill, I lost a lot of hair. I would wake up in the morning with a mat of hair on the pillow; when I washed my hair there were stringy clumps in my hands. After we moved to our clean house, my hair thickened and shed much less.

Starting around 2008, I had a condition called erythromelalgia. This is a rare disorder that causes pain, redness, and a burning sensation in the extremities, seemingly without any cause or trigger. For me, it was the feet—most frequently, one toe in particular. For years, I called it "rotten toe syndrome." For the two years I was the most ill, it came and went with my menstrual cycle. As I began to recover my baseline health, the erythromelalgia got worse, to the point that I had trouble walking and needed to wear loose sandals with socks when I went outside in winter. It felt like the affected toes were infected, rotting, and trying to heal themselves, all at the same time. Sometimes the pain spread to all of my toes. Doctors I saw at the time couldn't diagnose it, and I didn't insist because I had largely given up involving them in what I considered minor symptoms (like being hobbled).

I got chilblains. Chilblains are damage to flesh triggered by exposure to cold ambient temperatures, resulting in burning pain and sometimes open sores. My exposures to cold weather didn't seem severe enough to reasonably trigger the chilblains, so they are an indication of how messed up my body was. The medical literature doesn't make a connection between erythromelalgia and chilblains, but the symptoms are quite similar. The chilblains were most severe when the erythromelalgia was also at its worst. I only got chilblains on my hands, not my feet. During one winter, I had open sores and later scarring on the backs of all my fingers. I didn't see any doctors for the chilblains, which is bizarre to me now, but my inaction was a reflection of how demoralized and alienated I felt after earlier doctors' visits. I was able to self-diagnose the condition and knew that it would heal in time anyway. It wasn't as scary as the erythromelalgia, which didn't have any logic or healing timeframe to it.

For a few summers, I got spontaneous painful open sores on my arms if I was in the sun for more than a few minutes. The sores would appear rather quickly, and later they would heal and form little scars. Sometimes I only got the precursor burning feeling and no open wound. Probably this was a mild case of one of those rare autoimmune disorders in which the different layers of skin attack each other, like complex regional pain syndrome (CRPS). It was never diagnosed in my case.

This next is gross, but during these years I had a lot of thick, stinky, foul-tasting mucus, like a post-nasal drainage. I think this was a response to different environmental stimuli. I have noticed a connection between exposures to dust and this mucus, and I have also noticed a connection between commercial toothpaste in a tube and this mucus. I suspect other triggers but have been unable to identify them. Nasty.

A few years ago, for about six months, I had episodes of emotional lability, meaning socially inappropriate and uncontrollable expressions of laughter in my case. It only happened when we had company over or were visiting someone. I didn't then know what it was, but to myself I called it "the greeting disorder," like when a dog gets too overexcited around people. I have since learned that this condition is called pseudobulbar affect and that it is caused by neurological diseases or brain injury. When it happened to me, I felt happy, like a lonely dog who has received a visit, and would laugh for several minutes with tears running down my cheeks. Mostly the people around me took it well, although Husband did look concerned a few times.

I have low physical stamina and trouble building stamina. My parents and siblings are all marathoners and triathletes, and I jogged for many years. But I wasn't able to achieve true comfort while jogging, and it didn't get easier despite my determination. Now it is clear my basic physical health had been damaged from the beginning in a way that regular running could not correct.

I feel slight shame describing these various conditions, especially the revolting ones and the behavioral ones. But I do want to be as helpful as I can to other people and to tell the full truth about what happened to me.

# Chapter 32 - Pookie as Faust

Perhaps the greatest gift is knowledge bestowed to help the recipient. Sharing what you know is a powerful human motivation, and people especially want to help their loved ones with their own wisdom. Yet my mother and father, a psychologist and a history professor respectively, did not manifest this impulse with respect to me. It just wasn't there.

Throughout my teens and twenties, I was confused when I thought about the members of my family. I had deep faith in them, and I wasn't able to reconcile their negligence and abuse with my strong belief system. I told myself these events were based on misunderstandings and happened for mysterious reasons that I was not yet old enough or wise enough to understand. According to my internal logic, when I became older and more of a true person, less of the little shit that some members of my family told me I was, I would understand why these people, who were basically on my side, did what they did. I felt sad and a bit injured but was sure that through my hard work and good intentions I could accommodate whatever injuries I had suffered. If I had embraced the evidence in front of me, our family would have been blown apart and I would have been left with nothing.

If I summon a random memory of the family all together, say at the dinner table, Dad is grandstanding about some aspect of his job, his art collections, his investments, or his athletic prowess. Mom is looking down and away with her smile muscles slightly contracted but no joy on her face. The children are quiet and along for the ride. Mom and Dad did not discuss matters of importance when we were present. We children received an impression of private conversations and, in front of us, either implicit understanding and agreement between the two of them or Mom's silent compliance with Dad's decisions. Now I see that it was their secrets that prevented them from entering dialogues of unconditional sharing with us, from teaching us about the world and our potentials within it.

The exception was my mother toward my older sister. While Mom and Dad were the obvious, sanctioned, and unquestioned alliance, Mom and Kirsten formed a secret, forbidden alliance. Returning to this random memory of the family, I discern that Kirsten is not just along for the ride. While the three youngest children bounce around in the turbulence and unpredictability of Dad's alternating charisma and ill humor, she alone can quietly watch the adults and analyze the interactions between family members. She is safe because she has a secret protector.

Mom deliberately split the family into power centers to determine her own emotional destiny. She controlled Dad by helping him decide what he thought and did about his children, and she controlled Kirsten by forming Kirsten's views about the family and the world from an early age. Choosing certain family members over others is the strategy of a weak, diminished, and desperate person, not a large-hearted and generous person. Although Mom gained enormous power, it was a mean-spirited, selfish, and corrupting power, wielded against the meek and utterly defenseless. What did she see coming down the pike? She excluded three—we were the lost souls, left to make our own way in a brutal world, scrabbling against the odds to assemble the components of a meaningful life.

When I was young, I knew Mom and Dad had secrets, but I also knew these secrets were none of my business. Out of respect for their private lives, I deliberately avoided consideration of the various signs and signals that might have alerted me to the nature of their hidden truths. Now, fifty years later, I am revising my approach. What if their core secret was the lie they told about how I became ill as an infant, and their tendency to discuss important matters only in private was a habit that came from hiding this one big lie?

Taking this a step further, what if my early injury sowed the seeds that initially hobbled and later devastated the family? I don't want to be at the center of this disaster, but what if I am?

My parents were not born monsters. How do two middle-class people, academics and scientists who have the world as their oyster, teach their children nothing, feed and clothe them badly, and undermine their children's opportunities to build productive lives? What was the real reason they threw me away when I was fifteen? As I faced the two of them across the table during the legal deposition, I saw two people devoid of conscience, empathy, or filial impulses—two people determined to do maximum damage to protect themselves from exposure. Out of habitual deference, I did not acknowledge what I saw.

When I was in my teens and twenties, I wasn't capable of trading all I valued, meaning my love for my family, in exchange for true understanding of the world and my place in it. Now, the neurological trauma of my terrible illness has forced me into a Faustian bargain: clarity of thought and mental health in exchange for a full acknowledgment of the weakness and maybe even evil in the people I loved.

I've never liked my third-grade school picture. Each of the previous two years shows a pretty child wearing a fitted jumper with a sweet, collared white shirt underneath. When I was five and when I was six, my hair was evenly cut and the front bangs were pulled to one side and gathered into a small elastic, forming a tiny ponytail at one temple. I have good skin color and a responsive, engaged face. When I was seven and in the third grade, I wore for my school picture a way-too-big sleeveless dress that appears in an earlier photo on Kirsten. Kirsten wore it with a cute collared white shirt underneath, but I don't have a shirt underneath the dress and my arms look thin in the large armholes. The dress bags with folds across my chest, and the stitched-on daisies, needing ironing, sag and droop. My hair is uneven and there is no barrette or elastic. But it isn't just my clothes and hairstyle. I have sallow skin, shadows under my eyes, and an open-mouthed expression that is a cross between a gasp and a poor attempt to smile. I always tucked this photo underneath others. Surely I was not that ugly child, I told myself, until now.

Finally I look unblinking at the photo, and, with deep empathy and sadness, I recognize on my own face the same worried expression that the LTC actuaries had, back in the toxic workspace that made me so very ill. This was not a child who photographed badly on that particular day. This child was not ugly; she was ill. For years, I was repelled by this image because a deep truth resonated within me—an unwanted memory of a diminished and unloved self.

There is no way for me to know what the triggering exposure was, but I now believe that when I was in the third grade my parents became aware that I was again ill. They made the connection back to my neurological collapse as a baby, and it is hard to imagine the full nastiness of the shock they must have had when they realized they had not escaped that early horror. It is not possible to think well of yourself after learning that you have destroyed the health of your child. This shock ravaged my mother and then bound the two of them, corrupted, to each other. The timing is right. It was around then that Dad began hitting us too hard and without apparent reason. It was around then that Mom cut off her hair and stopped shaving her legs and buying new underwear. It was around then that Kirsten's bullying stepped up, and around then that, basically, our family turned to garbage.

Thirty years after the deposition, I do think their guilt and my mother's emotional withdrawal are enough to explain their treatment of me, who was an innocent among them. I don't believe there was more to their story or that there were other secrets of any significance. These were not complicated people. There isn't any more wisdom that I've got coming, and I'm not a little shit anymore. The early damage done to me was the hidden determinant of their adult lives, separately and together. This was the horrific revelation that my mother saw coming down the pike, against which she, with the complicity of the crap man who was her husband, twisted and corrupted our family.

# Chapter 33 - Revenge on Mom

~~

I deserve revenge on my mother, but I feel sorry for her and don't want her to suffer. She is a second child like me, and our natures are shaped by a deep desire to be better than others. My mother identified so strongly with Kirsten that she was made miserable by my beauty, both inner and outer. My husband also has inner and outer beauty, kind of off the charts. So maybe my revenge will be to become the person I was always meant to be, with my large and sweet-natured man beside me (naked). I think there will be more, though, and this is how it will happen.

Amy's baby teeth came in with thin and weak enamel. Poor childhood nutrition often causes this condition, and it's true we were not fed well because Dad didn't like spending money on groceries. So Amy's teeth were irregular and discolored, and she endured probably dozens of cavities before her adult set grew in. In a family photo when she was seven, she is wearing a way-too-large halter top, which I had sewn for myself but judged too weird to wear, and the same pair of red polyester bell-bottom pants that appears on her in other group photos around that time. She is tiny. Her hair was obviously cut by Dad. Despite these sartorial deficiencies and her mouthful of rotten stumps, she stands as straight as a goddess in ancient Egypt, staring at the camera with a level, clear-eyed gaze. She knew she was going to be somebody.

When I was fifteen to eighteen and Amy was ten to thirteen, she was struggling. Our parents ignored her except for Dad's criticisms of her character and ethics. She was disconnected and withdrawn and hadn't learned who she could be or how to make her way in the world. I thought that through infusions of understanding and caring I could help her become whole, and these impulses guided my behavior toward her for the next thirty years.

Once when I was fifteen and she was ten, Amy stole something from me or rifled my things—I forget exactly what happened. According to the family culture, I was supposed to hit her. I looked into her enormous blue eyes and at her creamy, beautiful little face and just couldn't do it. I felt like a failure and sensed that my weakness would render me susceptible to exploitation in the future. As I quivered before her skinny, badly dressed body, she looked unblinking back at me. She read on my face the life lesson that when weak people love you, you can take tangible and intangible goodies from them for as long as they have something that you want. Mom and I have in common our competitive natures, and we were also complete patsies when it came to Amy's thievery. As she stole from us and we refused to acknowledge it, we taught her who she could be and how to make her way in the world.

After I left for college, Amy wrote me and told me of a recent visit with Dad to the Waffle House. She drew a little picture of a tombstone with "RIP Amy" on it and lightning bolts exploding all around it. I imagined she might move to Cambridge to live with me, who loved her. I wrote in my journal, "Wonder if Amy and I could live together and what we would do with each other and to each other or if we would just rip each other apart." Many years later when she and her then husband were considering where to settle and raise their family, I wanted them to live near me, but she moved back to Hometown instead.

Amy was no fool. She had seen that when Kirsten and I were living together, Mom bought Kirsten clothes, got her a job, and took her out for lunches. Now, as a young adult and with a growing family, Amy attached herself to Mom and the free childcare, mortgage co-signs, and other weighty assistance Mom could give. She got an advanced degree in psychology like Mom, joined Mom's counseling and consulting partnership, gradually nudged out the other partners, and piggybacked on Mom's professional relationships to build her own career.

I frequently find jewelry and other oddments while walking down the street. In the summer of 1979, when my mother drove to Mexico with the three children who wanted to go, we visited the large Mesoamerican complex of pyramids outside Mexico City. In a pile of rocks off a path, I found a ceramic head about an inch high, from around 200 CE. No need for modern curios from the local market! I put it in my pocket then and still have it today. My point is that my subconscious peripheral vision used to be exceptional.

When Dad took the family to the beach or later when I went with my friends, I spent most of every day searching for fossilized shark teeth. I had an uncanny gift for finding them. With the logic of a child, I saw that because I was gifted and lucky, these beautiful objects came to me. The more of them I found, the better I was than other people. I learned which patches of shells (by their configuration and overall texture), which sections of beach, and what recent tidal activity and weather patterns were likely to yield the highest volume of these treasures. By their hues and outlines, they popped into my vision from among all the black, gray, and pinkish-gray shell fragments washed up on the sand. My siblings collected them not at all, or at least not directly from the sea, probably because I was so preternaturally skilled that they didn't want to enter the arena. I found quarts and quarts of them in total over the course of my life, in all sizes including tiny.

When I was forty-eight, I made a few passes through my possessions as I prepared for . . . what, exactly? From childhood I had accumulated treasures, and I wanted to find homes for my jewelry, my artifacts, and my small items of vintage material culture, whether purchased or found. My debilitation made me want to travel lightly toward the next phase, whatever it looked like. While I was doing a survey with deaccessioning in mind, I came across a couple of tablespoons of shark teeth in a small glass jar, along with some shells and beach glass. Where were the rest of them? I hadn't focused on the stash recently if ever. I generally took them home from the beach and then forgot about them. Then, not so much actual memories as remembered impressions came to me of missing things—mostly missing jewelry, but also shark teeth, missing by the handful over the years.

When I was a teenager, I knew Amy stole from me. Just as Mom did when Amy stole coins from her briefcase and later bills from her wallet, I pushed the knowledge aside. I felt sorry for Amy and didn't mind much. I had so many treasures, as well as jobs that earned me money to buy new ones, and I got used to a certain erosion of stock over the years. I didn't know how to talk to her about it and didn't want unpleasantness since she took criticism badly. When I was fifteen at Governor's School or seventeen at college, I would come home and things would be missing. I would feel sad for a minute and then be distracted by other aspects of my life.

By the time we were adults in our twenties, I assumed it had stopped. She visited regularly over the years, and I thought nothing of leaving her alone in my home. Then, with both of us in our forties, holding this little glass jar with a few dozen shark teeth rattling around in it, I had the full and conscious knowledge that she had never stopped stealing from me. The last time I handled this jar, maybe a few years before, there had been more of them. I knew she hadn't kept them but had thrown them away, and I would never get them back. She wanted to steal what was precious to me, even if she had no use for the pilfered objects.

I made a connection to the few times I deliberately ignored when she found ways to call attention to her breasts or lady parts in front of my boyfriends. She didn't want sex with these men; she wanted to see if she could take something valuable away from me. I remembered things she said about other family members that lowered my opinions of them, and I knew in that moment that she had said damaging things about me to my mother, my father, our other siblings. My sister wanted to hurt me, I realized, and it wasn't a pretty thing to learn. No wonder I put this knowledge off as long as I could. It was only the desperation and clarity that came from my life-threatening illness that allowed me to see this deeply unpleasant truth.

Amy had often looked at me with an even stare, and I realized she had been assessing the level of love coming from me so that she could ratchet up the thieving and associated carnage to match. I was horrified and ashamed—horrified at her inner nature, finally revealed to me, and ashamed of my denial of facts right in front of me for decades. I was a clueless mug, a sucker, an idiot.

∞

Several years have passed since then. Amy told her husband she wanted a divorce just a few months after insisting he get a vasectomy. I see this as her attempt to circumscribe his life so that in the future his resources would flow to herself and her children rather than to a new family. She had a virulent cancer and then a double mastectomy, and she reconstructed her breasts from her own fat. Both of her children have had serious asthma since early infancy, probably from the enormous and stench-ridden new cars that she buys. She now has the good hair, the good clothes, the good teeth.

Amy encouraged Mom to divorce Dad, and now I wonder if she did this because she knew Dad did not intend to pass wealth to his daughters. If Mom and Dad were together and Mom died first, Mom's wealth would go to Dad, and Amy would end up receiving very little. On the other hand, if they divorced and Mom died, Amy would get a great deal. After Mom settled the divorce from Dad and received her portion of accumulated assets, including art, Amy moved Mom into a house right across the street from herself. Husband and I imagined Amy lugging a European nineteenth-century bronze athlete or blacksmith back to her own house after every visit to Mom.

There has been plenty of time for me to reflect and remember since I noted with shock my meager tailings of shark teeth. I have become afraid of her. If she and I were put in a gladiator arena, I would turn and run to snatch a few more seconds of life before I felt her teeth in the back of my neck.

For many years I fancied I had saved Amy. As a young teen when she was neglected and withdrawn, Dad complained to me that she had no conscience, and I thought through my love I could give her one. What I did instead was teach her how to read the love and forgiveness on people's faces and then gain power by manipulating them, lying to them, and stealing from them.

But sometimes what goes around does come around. I loved her for many years, during which she was a joy and consolation to me, and now for the price of a gallon of ancient bone shards,

I am free of someone who would have sucked me dry if we lived nearer each other. Who is she sucking dry instead? Passive, generous, patient, and desperate for the redemption of a happy family after the mess she and Dad made of their own, Mom showers Amy with goodies and has done so for years. Mom has been writing the checks to Amy; paying for travel and meals out; running the errands; offloading her friends, her husband, and her colleagues; and handing over fistfuls of cash, divorce-settlement art treasures, her heart, maybe even her soul.

It won't be my spinal cord that will be severed by Amy's polished teeth; it will be Mom's. Will Mom realize what she has been harboring before she dies? Just as I went after Amy with my eyes wide open and pushed from me the neon-bright evidence of her true nature, Mom wanted what Amy offered: humor, acceptance, companionship, the illusion of family love. Perhaps it will be the approach of death that will help Mom see Amy with clarity, as it did for me. I didn't plan this revenge, but with some ambivalence and from a distance I can sense it unfolding.

# Chapter 34 - Disgruntlement

By early 2015 I had been at InsCo for fourteen years, six of them managing the finance function in the small RINS business unit. I had worked from home exclusively for about three years, the last year and a half from the other side of Massachusetts. After ParCo acquired InsCo in 2004, shareholder and market pressures to cut expenses led to paroxysms of consolidation, meaning layoffs combined with organizational restructuring. The most recent, still ongoing across the company, involved moving the finance functions out of the individual business units and into centralized finance service centers. Many of my long-term colleagues at larger business units were laid off. Some scrabbled for diminished positions at InsCo, and many disappeared.

I imagined that due to the complexity of the RINS finance function and the long tenure of its staff, upper management realized it was cheaper to leave such deep expertise in place. But I was wrong. In prior years I had repeatedly asked for new projects and volunteered for work outside my usual job functions. To the wrong-minded, these offers meant I was underemployed. Several years earlier I had raised objections with my then supervisor and also with HR to the frequent sexual innuendos made by the head of the business unit. These objectionable comments stopped abruptly and completely after my interference. I did this man a favor by retraining him, but eventually he figured out I was behind his HR drubbing and held a grudge. Due to waves of restructuring in the echelons above our business unit, I had had five supervisors during a period of five years. Because my supervisors were short-term, there wasn't anyone who knew the true measure of my contributions. Also, my illness meant I was unable to maintain a personal presence within the ever-changing leadership structures. Probably my work-from-home status was vaguely associated with malingering. For all of these reasons, in early 2015 and via conference call, I learned from my two most recent supervisors—one of whom happened to be sexual-innuendo Dude; the other I will call Stina—that my group would be eliminated and myself and all but one of my staff would be severed. Dude and Stina expressed their intentions to do whatever they could to help me find another suitable position within the company.

Initially, I was to stay for two months to train my replacements, but as the implementers of the transition learned more about the scope of my job, they extended the time. They extended it again to a total of eight months, which was through the end of December. If I left on my own accord before the severance date they chose, even as that date changed, I would lose important benefits.

My last eight months at InsCo ended up being a rollercoaster of sweet successes and bitter disappointments. During the transition of my responsibilities to the new service centers, most of the people I worked with were acquaintances rather than long-term colleagues. These people were professional and pleasant because they needed important information about how I did my job, but they didn't make the effort to invest in a relationship because I would soon be gone. After my long time in the corporate world, I had low expectations for emotional gratification. I wasn't bothered by these people.

I was not fine, however, with events and management decisions that indicated a deeper selfishness and disregard. Some of these events and decisions were initiated by me and some evolved because of my illness and historical personal relationships, but, regardless of the source, all this drama helped me to finally see the company clearly. I understood that I had not been treated well and that the company's purported corporate culture was a lie. I also saw that because of the circumstances surrounding my illness, I had become a dumping ground for unfair and unethical decisions. My sense of injustice grew. By the end I was seething with lava pits of burning malice and disgruntlement, thinly crusted over. The various reasons for my disgruntlement are important because of the large and delicious revenge-based action I took after my last day.

I love that word, *disgruntled.* It reminds me of the dwarf named Grumpy but suggests that the attitude is not self-adopted but is inflicted by outside forces. I had been a bit disgruntled even before being severed because one of my five recent supervisors was a vicious bully. After this nasty man left the company abruptly, I had occasion within the upward-feedback mechanism to refer to him as "a workplace-bullying lawsuit waiting to happen." Probably my bluntness on this occasion was yet another reason upper management did not see me as a keeper.

After I first got the news that I would be laid off, I hoped management would change its mind and keep me on in some capacity. I also wanted to maintain my self-image as ethical, competent, and professional and wanted my colleagues to remember me that way. Without kissing anyone's ass and while standing firm when necessary, I was supremely helpful and showed enormous strategic initiative to successfully transition my work to the new groups—kind of like a pig gathering sticks for the smokehouse fire. I received slights and disappointments, some small and some large, that caused me to become angry even as I wanted to stay.

When Dude and Stina said they would do whatever they could to help me find another job within the company, which was my best shot at continued employment given the severity of my disability, I didn't believe they intended to do much. They ended up doing nothing, and I felt disrespected by their lies. I tried to find jobs for my staff within the organizational structures of these two people and had no luck, even though my proposals were completely workable. I suggested to sexual-innuendo Dude that I stay on part-time and at a reduced job grade to perform a particularly complex reconciliation function that I knew he would have trouble accomplishing without my expertise. He turned me down. Stina was well-placed to help me find another job but had no incentive to do so since I was most useful in my current position helping her with the transition of my work. I applied for many suitable jobs within the company with no luck, and in some of these cases I sensed Stina's hand. To her, I was chum, not as in a good friend, but as in dead fish parts floating in deep water.

There was zero effort on my behalf from HR. InsCo was downsizing its population of staff at my level and replacing us with younger, cheaper folks, but during those eight months there were still many suitable jobs posted, and I had always received favorable performance reviews. The company had loudly championed its culture of staff development, but evidently these were empty words since managers did not believe a long-time employee was a worthy hire. I wrote to vice presidents of my acquaintance asking for a job but sensed that my philosophy of helping others to be successful in their jobs whenever possible had been seen as accommodating femininity rather than an indicator of leadership.

In hindsight, I'm happy the job disappeared from my life, but at the time I was devastated. I had Stockholm syndrome, in which a captive loves and reveres her captor. As I was repeatedly rejected, this strong attachment gradually changed to schadenfreude and the desire to cause a lot of trouble.

The groups taking on my team's work had to staff up well beyond their initial calculations because splitting up the complex work we had done was far less efficient than doing it all in one place. I felt vindicated and overjoyed as I watched this unfold. Ultimately, nine staff equivalents were needed to replace my team of five. The cost of this permanent increase was on top of training the new staff and fixing their mistakes. In the end, after about a year of planning and execution involving dozens of people, the company had offloaded an efficient and high-performing team whose average tenure was twelve years and who were not overpaid, and replaced it with almost double the staff.

I saw a chance for revengement against sexual-innuendo Dude.

When I first started at RINS, I worked a lot with the "administration" area. This group was headed by a hardworking fellow who had bowel cancer. He was rigged up with a device or had some sort of sphincter weakness that caused frequent loud flapping noises from his nether regions. He apparently had no control over these emissions, which I thought would have been enough to keep him at home. We were all supposed to ignore the alarming sounds, I suppose, and initially I felt kindly toward him. Our job functions should have made us natural allies, and we both had strong technical expertise and competence with computer systems, but he was suspicious and unhelpful. I tried for years to achieve a deep reconciliation of our respective data systems to explain a stubborn variance of about $1.2 million, but he stonewalled at every opportunity, discounted my concerns to sexual-innuendo Dude, and turned his staff against me. I started calling him Farter Phil to my husband.

Farter Phil died a few years later. I continued to try to get this $1.2 million variance resolved. I produced Herculean volumes of deep analysis and documentation but did not get the support I needed from Farter Phil's replacement or sexual-innuendo Dude. I felt that these men discounted my concerns mostly because of my gender.

When I was to be severed and outsiders became involved, I highlighted the missing $1.2 million and mentioned "potential fraud," knowing full well these words were incendiary. Publicly traded companies suffer severe reputational damage if it becomes known that they ignored employees reporting missing assets. As fuel, I provided several memos and emails, dated at approximate yearly intervals, which documented my continual efforts to resolve the problem and which were addressed to Farter Phil and sexual-innuendo Dude. Sexual-innuendo Dude was raked over the coals for ignoring my warnings and requests for help, and two internal fraud investigators drove two hours from Boston to interview me for a day. Teams of people came to RINS in Boston from the ParCo mother ship to understand our processes and systems. As they scrambled to develop missing expertise, I flaunted my raw talent for complex forensics and reconciliations. I knew that however helpful I was and however many bodies they threw at this problem, they were going to struggle mightily to resolve it.

I didn't have and didn't express an opinion as to whether or not Farter Phil stole the money, but I had a massive volume of historical forensics to prove he could have. As I pointed out, he was dying for a long time, the timing was right, he had the necessary access to the financial systems and cash-payment processes, he was concerned about the financial well-being of his family, and he obstructed my efforts to resolve the issue at every turn, including undermining my reputation to his staff and the head of the business unit.

At each stage of this investigation, I was thrilled at the amount of work it was causing other people and overjoyed at the mortification of my enemies. I was not privy to the end result, but the investigation was heading toward the deeply embarrassing conclusion of probable fraud. There was a delicious postscript to this embezzlement imbroglio. A few months after I left, the younger, cheaper person to whom I had transitioned my reconciliations and forensics expertise transferred to a new job within the company, effectively rubbishing the massive investment that had been made in him.

Anticipating that I might be unemployable, I filed for workers' compensation benefits. This state-regulated insurance provides support for those who are injured at work, which had obviously happened to me in 2010. Although I had had responses to environmental toxins before 2010, the LTC workspace had disabled me.

My initial filing was erroneously marked as closed. I refreshed the claim and was interviewed for fifteen minutes over the phone by an insurance-company examiner. She rejected the claim using vague explanatory language. I wrote emails to five people within the company who were familiar with my injury, telling them the key issues they should address when the workers' compensation examiner contacted them. I got an email from an HR hack telling me not to contact anyone in the company about my claim. I put together an enormous package of documentation including medical records, emails to my supervisors back in 2010, write-ups explaining the sequence of events with specific dates of injury, and the years-long documentation of my environmental exposures and symptoms. I included my list of five witnesses and copies of the emails I had sent them. The insurance company rejected me again, and I was able to determine that they had not contacted any of these five people. I pressed on and ultimately received a final denial citing "prior diagnosis," meaning that somewhere in my medical records prior to 2010 a doctor had diagnosed chemical intolerance. I was enraged. Symptoms of chemical intolerance were nowhere in my medical records prior to mid-2010, and there wasn't even a tentative diagnosis until 2013. This workers' compensation insurance system clearly possessed a profoundly unfair bias in favor of the insurers and the company, neither of whom were acting in good faith. This was not a benefit that I had available, and I felt disrespected and lied to. Employees, beware: this particular system is rigged against you.

There were hundreds of individual tasks that needed to be transferred away from my group. During December, the new owners of these tasks dramatically increased the urgency and frequency of their requests for meetings and ad hoc guidance. The company was apparently committed to a firm last day for me, and I knew why. Bonuses for a calendar year are paid at the end of February of the following year. This cash serves as an incentive for staff who might otherwise leave the company to stay through the complex grind of the year-end accounting close process, while working overtime for free. If InsCo kept me past December, they would have had to keep me through February for the close, admit the defeat of their transition timetable, and pay me a bonus of around $25,000. It was cheesy to put on so much pressure during my last month just to prevent me from earning a bonus.

And there was a bigger financial loss, as I saw it. Since I had worked for the company for fifteen years, I should have gotten thirty weeks of severance pay. But in 2011 my tenure had been interrupted when I had had to leave because of illness, so the first eleven years did not count. The interruption of less than a month was due to my illness from the workspace, as I explained to HR and my supervisors. No luck. I sensed that sexual-innuendo Dude was the primary decider in this case. Providing I dutifully signed a standard release of claims agreement, and initially I saw no reason not to, I was to receive a fairly modest severance payment considering my long service. The difference was around $50,000.

Sometimes people get so caught up with kicking someone else in the teeth that they lose perspective. They make decisions that reflect deeper selfishness and ethical deficits than they normally allow themselves. This is what had happened to sexual-innuendo Dude. The decision to pay the lower severance amount wasn't reasonable under the circumstances. Perhaps the fact that I had filed a workers' compensation claim, however fact-based the claim, helped him justify this unfairness.

Although I was happy to have my salary continue for the full eight months, these aspects of my treatment, as well as older disappointments, ratcheted up the rankle factor. With the fraud investigation and the doubling of staff assigned to my work, I had gotten a taste of sweet revenge. I dreamt of further damage I could do to InsCo, within the law.

# Chapter 35 - Big Cool Friend

It is hard to take control of a relationship in which you have long been powerless and to rebel against conventional strictures of loyalty and the desire for approval. When we enter the corporate world, we naturally align our interests with those of the corporation that gives us so much. The more we believe in the benevolent intentions of our employer, the more rewarding is our work and therefore also our lives. I worried about what ex-colleagues would say about me, and I worried about unspecific acts of retribution. But whenever I thought of hurting the business unit and the company badly, I felt a surge of excitement and joy. It was this exhilaration that made me overcome my fears, gird my lions (I do mean large cats), and take direct action.

The leaders of this company value profits. To hurt them, you must cost them money. The ideal is to cost them a truly vast sum of money through a process that requires large administrative effort and therefore expense. If, at the same time, they suffer embarrassment from reputational risk, you achieve an ethical triumph, and you get some cash, then fan-tastic.

I would need a big cool friend who was prepared to do the heavy lifting.

The IRS whistleblower webpage explains how it works. First, you as a virtuous citizen send them information about a specific instance of tax evasion or tax exploitation. If the IRS deems your story credible and worth the effort, they will pursue audit, enforcement, and collection of the tax deficiency plus any interest and penalties due. The process will take many years, but they will send you a hefty percentage of the total amount they ultimately collect. After scanning the webpage, I sat back and considered from different angles the Barbados tax wheeze that I resented so deeply and that had damaged my career prospects years before.

Because of my anxious state, I found the IRS website terrifying at first. Rather than engaging with their forms and process directly, I looked for help online. Some law firms specialize in whistleblower claims, and I picked one based on their website graphics. I started a conversation with them about their terms of engagement were they to help me file the claim. This firm was located in a large city in California, and I imagined glass-walled conference rooms with long vistas. Per telephone conversation, they would help me for 30 percent of the amount that the IRS awarded to me. If the IRS awarded me nothing, they got nothing. But after a few phone calls and emails and after getting a draft engagement contract from them, I became afraid of the whistleblower lawyers. I worried that despite the contingency arrangement, the convoluted language of the agreement allowed for a nightmare scenario in which I owed them a lot of money I didn't have.

They didn't express an interest in my legal exposure under the terms of the employment contract or the release of claims severance agreement, either for my disclosure of company information or for anything else. I thought that advice regarding risk to myself should be part of their service, but it became clear they saw me as raw meat only. Yes, they had experience with similar IRS claims, but I didn't need their experience to succeed with my claim. I didn't see the point of being involved with them if I then had to hire a second tranche of lawyers to advise me on risk exposure. The naked greed of these predators frightened me, and I offloaded them.

Although these people scared the shit out of me, I did learn from the growing vigor of their pursuit of me that they felt my potential claim had merit. They told me they had hired a private investigator to research me personally and had evidently found me credible, which meant the IRS would as well. As I assessed the risks and potential success of an IRS whistleblower claim, these indications were encouraging.

There were further concerns. One was the aforementioned disclosure of company information. Could InsCo sue me for providing data about their business to the IRS? I looked first to the employment contract I signed when rejoining the firm after my extreme illness. The relevant language was fairly vague. It referred to a relationship of confidence and that I was not to disclose any proprietary or confidential information. I arranged for a brief telephone consultation with a lawyer who advised that the term "confidential information" was a term of art, meaning that it was open to interpretation based on factors like the degree of secrecy and protection surrounding the data.

Any information I was considering providing to the IRS had been widely known both within and outside of the business unit and was not password protected. In town hall meetings, sexual-innuendo Dude repeatedly crowed to the entire RINS staff about the huge tax savings achieved by the treaty with the ParCo Barbados affiliate. At no point were any aspects of the RINS business said to be confidential, and I had never received any training on how to treat confidential information.

My sharing of information with the IRS would be a good-faith disclosure in the interest of a wider ethical good, namely appropriate payment of taxes due the government. At one end of the scale is password protected, highly proprietary, and deeply secret information that is disclosed in order to damage a company's competitive position or for some other destructive purpose. At the other end of the scale is widely discussed information, available on computer servers to anyone within the entire division, that is disclosed in the interest of tax justice and to assist a government regulatory agency with its enforcement efforts. Clearly my situation exemplified the latter end of this scale. Therefore, I had nothing to fear from the confidentiality clause in the employment agreement.

Then I looked to the severance and release of claims agreement. It contained the same confidentiality clause, which was now not a concern, but it also contained language that I had waived all rights to recover money in connection with any charge, claim, or complaint filed with any administrative agency. If the IRS, an administrative agency of the US government, sent me money from the whistleblower claim and InsCo found out, they could force me to give it to them.

This was bad news. If I wanted cash today in the form of severance payments, I risked forfeiting whistleblower funds at a future date. Or did I? The company provided forty-five days after my date of severance to return the signed agreement. In the meantime, they commenced to pay me semimonthly severance benefits equal to my previous salary payments. Because of my illness and interrupted service, I was only to receive these severance payments for seven weeks—or, just over forty-five days! I could just do nothing and continue to receive the stream of direct-deposit amounts coded into their payroll computer systems. I checked with my bank on the ability of a payor to claw back a payroll deposit, which turned out to be a five-day window. It was unlikely that InsCo HR was on the ball enough to either interrupt the payment stream once it started or claw back the last payment, so I did not sign or return the release of claims.

The last payment came through and sat intact for five days. I was ecstatic over the success of my small gesture of rebellion. My joy came from taking a stand against an abusive and unfair agreement and also from signifying my intent to take further destructive action.

I filled out the form and put together an explanatory package for the IRS, including a detailed road map to the economics of the RINS business as well as to the wheeze treaty. I included extensive suggestions for the information requests that the IRS would need to make. Telling them what they would need to gather rather than providing these items myself further reduced my risk under the confidentiality clause of the employment agreement. RINS had never been part of the overall InsCo audit, meaning my claim would absolutely inform the IRS of an issue not previously on their radar screen. As I read through my package, which I did many times while practically slavering with happiness, I knew that any presentation by the scary whistleblower lawyers in California would not have been as good as the one I submitted myself.

If the company had agreed to give me the full thirty weeks of severance pay, I would have happily signed the release of claims agreement. I now realize that it would have been a strategic and ethical mistake to do so, but at the time I didn't see the situation as clearly as I do now. Back then, I would have been unwilling to give up the additional $50,000 for a tiny chance of getting a large amount of money many years in the future.

How much money are we talking about here? The insulting and ethically dubious decision to save $50,000 will end up costing InsCo at least $50 million. Past taxes saved, plus interest, plus an estimate for taxes they planned to save over the next few years, equals about $50 million. This is a low estimate because actually InsCo would cheat the US government out of $3 million a year forever if they could, not just for the next few years. The annual amounts were projected to increase by a large chunk in future years, and possibly InsCo will pay tax penalties if the scheme is determined to be utterly without merit (which it is). The real cost will be in the range of $100 million. Yaaaayyy!!! Now we're talkin'.

What will I receive? Hard to tell. I'm not sure how many of the treaty years the IRS will give me credit for, and my share will be between 15 percent and 30 percent. I certainly won't get paid for preventing future tax exploitation, only for tax abuse of the past. When overall settlements are negotiated for these years as part of audit horse-trading, the IRS may drop this issue in exchange for advantageous settlement on a larger issue or they may drop it for some other reason. I might get as much as $10 million, or I might get nothing.

Initially the chance of receiving money seemed so slight to me that the potential future payout was only a small reason for my action. I wanted to cause trouble and embarrassment and hopefully to cost InsCo a lot of money. Even if my bosses couldn't prove on paper who made the IRS suddenly pick up the Barbados wheeze as an audit issue, deep inside they would know I had achieved my revenge against all the odds, and they would know why I had done it.

At the time of my severance, I was so blinded by disgruntlement that I didn't have much room for ethical considerations. I now see my IRS whistleblower action as completely ethical and even a moral obligation, but over the previous years, I had gotten used to the wheeze. When you align your interests with those of your employer, their system of morality becomes yours, to some extent at least. As I prepared the package for the IRS, I had many imaginary conversations with angry ex-colleagues in which I tried to justify my decision. One minute, I felt guilty about the trouble these people would go through, and the next minute, I was elated at the trouble I was going to cause. Although I consider that I ultimately ended up in the right place, it was a struggle to get there. I hope to provide others the courage to take similar stands in the face of tax injustice.

If sexual-innuendo Dude had not wanted to get rid of me for speaking up years before about his ghastly comments about sex and women and had instead assessed with clarity my institutional knowledge and potential continued contributions to the company, I would still be employed and would never have filed the action. If the company had manned up and made an effort to find me another job in the light of my disability and long tenure or if they had considered my workers' compensation claim in a fair-minded and unbiased manner, I would never have filed the action. If they had not treated me so badly when I became ill in the workspace years before and had considered the full implications of a toxic space to all of their staff, I would not have become as angry as I did. Of course, at the root of it all is their own culture of tax exploitation. If they weren't so ethically bereft as to implement such a cynical and low-minded scheme in the first place, so arrogant as to imagine they would get away with it, and so disregarding of their staff as to not realize that their staff could easily report the wheeze, they wouldn't have exposed themselves to immense administrative expense, significant interest and penalties, and embarrassing ethical comeuppance.

# Chapter 36 - Stick, then Carrot

About a month after the hotly anticipated final severance payment came through, I received a telephone call from Julie, the HR flack who had been my contact for administrative issues during my last eight months there. Her name was all over the various official-looking documents regarding the terms of my end of employment. As a nostalgic gesture, I have a landline without caller ID, so I always have a little surprise when I pick up the phone. During the entire previous year, I had been in a state of general agitation, and I still had nervous excitement from sending the package to the IRS. I got a modest adrenalin shock and incipient drymouth when I realized who was on the phone.

Julie was calling about the release of claims agreement: did I remember it, and had I signed it? Yes, I said, I did remember it and I had not signed it. She said they had made a mistake and they should have stopped the severance payments since they had not received the signed agreement, implying by her tone that I had received some largish amount of money I wasn't entitled to. I said nothing, knowing full well the amount they could reasonably have stopped payment on was only one week's salary and also that there was no way they could claw it back. But her little exaggeration alerted me, never a quick thinker in conversation, that she was on a shit trick. After a little more back and forth, I explained that I was pretty ambivalent about signing it.

Julie brought out the big guns, "stick, then carrot" style. She said I was on a list to receive a bonus. She mentioned my two recent supervisors by name and said they had both forgotten to tell me about the bonus. She said the bonus had been inadvertently omitted from the letters I received about my severance benefits. She said it wasn't too late to receive the bonus if I returned the release of claims. She said I would get the bonus if I sent the signed release pretty soon, within the next few weeks, she thought.

I became instantly enraged; at the time I wasn't sure why the effect was immediate, but later I realized my insta-rage was due to the five lies right in a row. I said her news was completely unexpected and I had had no hint of this whatsoever in the many letters and memos I had received about my severance benefits. I became firm in my tone. She repeated a few more times that if I sent in the signed form by some uncertain date, I would get this bonus for the prior year. It would have been around $25,000. I repeated my surprise at the lack of documentation, implying disbelief, and allowed my tone to become slightly hostile. To get her off the phone, I said three times that I would think about it, and we rang off.

At InsCo, bonuses are one of the key ways for the company to control employee behavior. They are calculated as a percentage of annual salary, and tiny upward increments in this percentage are attributed to degrees of performance excellence. Looking back on the company's almost-annual overhauls of the reward infrastructure as they continually struggled with how to motivate folks effectively, it is laughable how small the differences were between rewards for mediocre work versus excellent work. The constants down the years were extreme specificity around who would get a bonus and tight budgeting control with many layers of review over the calculation of the amounts.

Based on my intimate understanding of the bonus calculation and granting processes, and the important leverage that bonuses gave to leadership, I knew it was impossible that I had been on a list to get one and not been told about it. My primary supervisor and I spoke many times a week during my last months at the company. She would never have forgotten about it since she absolutely would have used this information to control and motivate my behavior. It didn't ring true that there were mistakes made in the documents I received about my severance benefits. The company had been laying off staff for years, and, if true, their severance-related document templates would have contained options for post-severance payment of bonuses. These documents are extremely carefully vetted before being distributed, and it was deeply unlikely that this text was inadvertently left off my letters. Historically bonuses were only paid if the staff person was still employed at the end of February, and it had been clear to me during December that there was increased urgency to transition my work so that I would leave before the end of the year and not be owed one.

The last lie involved when I needed to send the form back to get the bonus. Julie was suspiciously vague, which told me she didn't have either the intention to pay or the actual funds lined up.

I couldn't believe this large company would allow their HR department to lie so outrageously to disadvantaged ex-employees. I was shaken by the utter cynicism of this call, and, for the next couple of weeks, I half expected to get an official letter laying out the terms of the "bonus for release of claims" exchange, with a firm due date. Such a letter would have meant that although I hadn't been on a list for a bonus, the company was still willing to pay me $25,000 for the signed release. This letter never arrived.

Probably Julie's supervisors maintained a spreadsheet listing the severed, with a checkbox next to each name. There was a green box if the signed form had come back and a red box if it hadn't. When they sat in weekly conference picking over the ashes and bone-chips of discarded long-term staff, they regarded the single red box next to my name with annoyance. They dangled a chunk of cash in front of me, assuming I would realize too late that I would never get it and that any attempt to enforce the promise was futile. There is a slim possibility that Julie was a rogue improvisor, but I don't think she had the humor or brains for that degree of creativity.

I considered: what would motivate them to tell so many egregious lies? It could only be the release of claims section that waived all rights to recover money in connection with a claim filed with a governmental administrative agency. They wanted to eliminate my financial motivation for filing an IRS whistleblower action. If by some chance I had already filed one, they wanted to establish a claim on my portion of a future settlement. This degree of strategic thinking was beyond Julie or her direct colleagues, which meant that the involvement of the real brains in the company, folks in corporate tax, had been triggered.

Based on my deep understanding of the culture and organizational structure and of the personalities within HR, the business unit, divisional management, and the corporate tax area, I can guess the sequence of events. This clumsy telephone call was the first delicious indication of their scrambling to contain the slow bleed of the RINS tax wheeze.

# Chapter 37 - The Slow Bleed

The IRS does not provide periodic updates on the status of a whistleblower claim. This is fair since InsCo tax issues are none of my business. The IRS will tell me if and when they have rejected my claim or if they have resolved the underlying tax issue without any payment due to me. Their website contains a flowchart with approximate time ranges for the stages of prosecution of a claim. This flowchart tells me that my claim has passed through the initial vetting stages and is now in the field-exam stage. I know intimately what this means from my prior experience in the corporate tax group at InsCo, where my primary responsibility was mid-level field-exam liaison to the IRS auditors.

A couple of weeks after I sent the package to the IRS whistleblower office in Ogden, Utah, I got a note that it had been received and was being processed. This was thrilling. Then, a couple of weeks later, I received a note that the claim had been forwarded to a different office where it would be coordinated in the future. My impression from the flowchart is that this new coordinating office is also home to the subject-matter expert for the technical nature of the claim; financial services, for example, or insurance. This was also thrilling. Just as I had for the first note, I studied the language for any hint of an underlying story. I tried to see behind the lines of text, into the IRS inboxes and conference rooms, to witness staff discussions regarding the likely viability of my claim. As of this writing, it has been two years since I received these notices. There has been nothing further, nor do I expect to receive any news for many years. Classic no news is good news. I will now imagine what happened since I left the company.

While my claim was being routed to the IRS subject-matter expert, HR staff responsible for tracking outstanding release of claims forms noted that mine had not been timely received. This noncompliance was discussed in a staff meeting as a cause for mild concern since nearly everyone who was laid off returned it. The fact that I hadn't returned it raised the possibility that I had a reason. HR staff then realized they should have turned off the paycheck spigot or made arrangements to claw back my last severance payment. They consoled each other since the over-payment was small, but they became defensive because of their mistake and therefore pissed off at me.

Because nonreceipt was so unusual, the issue was escalated to the local head of HR, who arranged a brief conference call with my last supervisor Stina and also the head of the business unit, sexual-innuendo Dude. "Based on your relationship with Pookie or her recent behavior," HR Head asked, "does this raise any red flags?" Dude said no, he didn't think so, since my behavior during my last eight months had been exemplary. He remembered me as being in shock when I first learned I would be severed, but shortly afterward I rallied and had many helpful suggestions while my work was being transitioned to the new groups. Stina agreed. I had never failed to pick up my phone during working hours and had shown unusual initiative in transitioning a great deal of complex work. HR Head pressed on, "Was there anything in her history?" Stina remembered there had been unusual circumstances surrounding the calculation of my severance period and that, due to interrupted service, the payment was much smaller than my long tenure indicated.

"Did she express bitterness over the lower amount?" HR Head made Dude and Stina dig deeper. It came out that I believed I had become disabled at work and that I had filed a workers' compensation claim that failed. Also, Dude admitted that many years earlier I had expressed repeated and heartfelt objections to an affiliate agreement because it was unjustified from a tax perspective. The allocated time for the conference call started to run out without a resolution, so another call was scheduled for the following week to which a few new players were invited.

One new player was Stina's boss George the Berator. George and sexual-innuendo Dude were at the same executive echelon and had hated each other for ten years. Recent organizational restructuring had thrown them together after they had been on separate paths for a while. George made up for the absence by heaping vitriol on Dude's head in front of other people at every opportunity, to the discomfiture of some and the amusement of the low-minded. The other two new players were the compliance officer for RINS and Tax Joe, the head of US Tax. HR Head sent a copy of the release of claims along with the conference call invite.

Before the second conference call, HR Head telephoned sexual-innuendo Dude for a private conversation about my complaints regarding his behavior years earlier. They relived Dude's most infamous comment, which was at an office Christmas party around 2012. (This is a true story.) There was a gift-exchange game going on, and about a hundred people watched as a RINS staff member with an enormous, noble, and improbably pointy bosom carried a wine-bottle rack to the front of the room to exchange it for something else. Probably most of the eyes in the room were on her bosom. Dude called out loudly that he did want the rack, but not the wine rack. In the ensuing appalled hush, another officer of the company said: "Where's HR when you need them?"

Dude assured HR Head that after being reprimanded, he completely cleaned up his behavior. He doubted I would be filing a sexual-harassment lawsuit. To frighten Dude into coming clean, HR Head went through her file containing the other comments and behaviors I had complained about. Dude squirmed. Of course he provided the same opportunities for advancement and the same rewards to men and women, he lied. He knew that such lawsuits require cash and an appetite for messy and humiliating prosecution, and women almost never pursue them. HR Head and Dude agreed to keep this aspect of my history a secret during the upcoming conference call.

Folks gathered for the second call. They developed the first dim collective awareness that they had exposure, which is business speak for "something bad could happen." HR Head, having considered the possible degree of disgruntlement from the unholy trinity of severance, disability, and ethical objection to tax wheeze, had reviewed the release of claims for potential areas of exposure. She went through a laundry list with the call participants. Did I possess proprietary competitive information that could damage RINS in the marketplace? No. Was there any other damaging use I could make of confidential information? No, the business unit didn't have information that could be deemed confidential. Was it likely I could disparage the company in a way that would be damaging? No, no one would listen to me. Were there any issues that could cause the company trouble with the SEC? No. The IRS? Ah—here there might be a problem, Tax Joe acknowledged.

In its sixty-plus years of existence, the business unit had never been in scope for the IRS auditors. This was because the business was small, it was unusually complex and hard to understand, it had been tucked away in a division separate from the rest of the US businesses, and the IRS had their hands full with large and typical investment and insurance tax issues, including the LILOs. In 2007, the implementers of the affiliate wheeze thought it was unlikely that the business unit would ever be audited. But if the attention of the IRS were drawn to the business unit and if they had a roadmap to its underlying economics, it would be apparent that the wheeze had no justification, Tax Joe acknowledged. George the Berator, whose twin philosophies for corporate success are "the best defense is a good offense" and "always carry a long knife," immediately began to abuse sexual-innuendo Dude for the treaty, even though George himself had been one of the original proponents. The call descended into a cacophony of recriminations and gibberish for a while, and, with time running out, everyone agreed to separately consider the points discussed and reconvene in a week.

In the meantime, Tax Joe called HR Head. If there was any way to get the form in, he said, it might yet prevent Pookie from filing a whistleblower action in the future. "She has only been gone for a couple of months, and she may not yet be aware of the possibility," he explained. Because Tax Joe is an extremely strategic person with a long view, he also realized that if I returned the form and then disregarded the confidentiality clause and filed a successful whistleblower claim, they could sue me for my own proceeds. This way InsCo could at least recover a largish portion of their payment to the IRS and poke a stick in my eye at the same time.

HR Head called Dude to brainstorm about how they might persuade me. They decided to use an implied threat that I needed to return the severance overpayment. If this insinuation didn't work, they would offer me a bonus and explain that due to an error I had not been notified that I was due for it. This was a believable story, and I was unlikely to have a good reason for keeping the form if I were offered $25,000, they reasoned. Then, Dude realized that expense approval protocols required George the Berator's approval for the actual payment. He knew George would make him grovel for it. He wanted to retrieve the form for free, hero-style. So he and HR Head didn't line up the funds. Both of them had long experience taking advantage of employees in situations that were open to interpretation, and the employees often did not fight back. They agreed that they would promise me a bonus if I sent the form by some vague future date. When they then reneged on the promise, there would be absolutely nothing I could or would do about it.

Julie called me per their instructions. This effort was not a success. The third conference call convened. HR Head and Dude glossed over the details of their attempt to get the form from me but did tell the rest of the group that I had not been receptive to persuasion. The others got an impression that the telephone call to me might have had aspects that were slightly unethical, but they let it pass. They all acknowledged that my shortened severance period meant that I had no incentive to return it, and also that the company no longer had any leverage over me. George berated sexual-innuendo Dude for not approving the longer severance period, despite George's awareness of this decision and nonintervention at the time. Other suggestions for pressuring me were put forward by members of the group and rejected by the compliance flack. Tax Joe reiterated that the tax issue had a good chance of being a bust under audit. George abused Dude again, lifting everyone else's spirits, and then they all rang off.

# Chapter 38 - The Field Exam

After my job ended I felt beat-up. Nevertheless, I put a résumé together and started applying for jobs online, disclosing fully that I could only work from home due to disability. Over a period of several months, I applied for several hundred suitable jobs from Maine to the mid-Atlantic states, figuring I could psych myself into enthusiasm if anyone were interested. It became clear that no one would hire me based on telephone contacts only, meaning I would have needed to rent a car to travel to an in-person interview. But rental cars reek of off-gassing plastics and fragranced cleaning products, as do most offices, so I would have been impaired and unable to speak normally if I had turned up. Also, executive recruiters were reluctant to shill me because I was damaged property, meaning disabled. However qualified I was and even if I fancied I was still employable, this job search was a bust.

Per the flowchart on the IRS webpage, it took about three months for them to move my whistleblower claim from their national-claim coordinators down to the local auditors. InsCo is always under audit, and the IRS has about five full-time staff permanently located within InsCo's corporate workspace. After my claim had been deemed credible and worth pursuing by the central office and then sent to the IRS auditors at InsCo, it was absorbed into the regular workflow of these long-term staff. They spend the most effort on the field-examination stage, in which they carefully prepare information document requests (IDRs) to gather necessary data. Then they propose adjustments to the tax amounts due. Sometimes these proposed adjustments are negotiated between the IRS and the company and then either reduced or dropped completely.

During the period I worked closely with the IRS auditors, which ended twelve years ago, I found them to be pleasant, highly intelligent, and hardworking. They were also patient and determined, for to execute that job well requires great powers of endurance. Most had been assigned to InsCo for many years and had developed deep technical expertise about the company's investments and products.

In my form for the whistleblower claim, I explained how I had become familiar with the tax issue I was reporting. I related my history working on the IRS audit while in the corporate tax group and spoke of my dismay at InsCo's more dubious tax positions. I mentioned my frustration at other staff who deliberately obstructed the progress of the hardworking auditors, and that I had loudly and repeatedly objected to the affiliate wheeze, damaging my career. I also noted that I had been disabled by a toxic workspace and had been laid off. I was speaking the truth and adding sufficient color for my story to be credible, but I also wanted the auditors to view me with sympathy. It is possible that some of the auditors I knew are still there. I liked these people. They will receive the roadmap I prepared for them and enjoy a frisson of recognition when they see my name. I savor the possibility that I am communicating with one of my old friends across a great distance.

The IRS whistleblower website explains that my identity will not be revealed to the taxpayer, so RINS staff will only be able to guess who blew the whistle on them. I will imagine how this happened.

A few months after they received the package from the national office, the on-site IRS auditors provided the first tranche of RINS IDRs to the InsCo audit coordinators. Because this small business unit was appearing for the first time as the subject of IRS interest and because of the relative volume of requests, Tax Joe's staff sent him an email that included scans of the IDRs. After taking in the email subject line "RINS Information Document Requests," he pushed his chair away from his desk and sat back for a minute. He then quickly scanned the IDRs and immediately grasped the truth behind them. I had filed an IRS whistleblower claim for the RINS Barbados wheeze.

Tax Joe took a moment to recall working together over the years as I moved to different departments within the company. He remembered cheerful and lucid correspondence, complex schedules, and issues resolved on time with no errors. He remembered that after I found out I was to be severed, I wrote to him asking for a job.

He leaned forward again and forwarded the email to sexual-innuendo Dude for discussion. On the surface, these first IDRs were not especially alarming. They were intended to gather general information about the business unit, and there was no particular focus on the Barbados treaty. Dude said to Tax Joe, "They won't be able to build a case with this. They have no idea about how the business works." Tax Joe ignored his reassurances. He immediately knew from the breadth of this first layer of inquiry that the IRS had settled in for the long haul.

Tax Joe's general attitude was win some, lose some. If sexual-innuendo Dude and his pissant business wriggled like a worm on a hook because they were going to lose a bundle, it wasn't his problem. He was not about to be blamed for it.

George the Berator and a couple of Tax Joe's high-level tax colleagues joined Dude and Tax Joe for a conference call. Dude initially downplayed the chance of IRS success and therefore the need to take specific action, but Tax Joe knew that the folks who run the company do not enjoy surprises. If the IRS assessed a large amount of tax and interest, this would affect reported company earnings. In fact, the tax area was obligated to enforce taking an adjustment to income immediately, according to their best guess of the ultimate amount due. Possibly there would also be reputation risk from the tax issue itself, since income shifting to tax-free jurisdictions did not play well in the press. Nothing made his bosses angrier than receiving sudden bad news they should have received the week before.

George berated sexual-innuendo Dude briefly but effectively, in front of the executive vice presidents, for allowing the circumstances to evolve that made me file the claim. The assembled group meditated briefly either on the loss of a talented staff member with deep institutional knowledge or how to cover their own asses in the coming shitstorm. In the end, Tax Joe was persuaded not to recommend an earnings hit to company leadership just yet.

In previous years, I would have cranked out the IDR responses by myself, but my group had been broken up and replaced by many remote service centers and none of them knew the business well. A cross-functional task force was established. During its weekly meetings, each member treated the open items as glue traps that they didn't want to touch. Because no one stepped up, arrangements were then needed for half of the time of a mid-level staff person to be allocated for the foreseeable future to interpret the requests, distribute them to the appropriate people for fulfillment, and then follow up repeatedly to enforce delivery.

At this stage, Dude made a strategic error. He mentioned to two RINS group leaders the suspicion that I was behind the leak. Because he had drunk his own Kool-Aid and because he habitually discounted women, he believed I had done something wrong, and therefore he was justified in complaining to folks not yet in the know. Hints got out into the wider RINS population that I had done something to hurt the company and that it had to do with the Barbados treaty. This rumor moved through the ranks and was reinforced by the numerous IDRs that went out to the people who had picked up my work.

It is not good for a company if one of its severed staff makes a mint reporting the company's misdeeds to the government. It becomes worse if other staff find out. They might view the ex-employee with sympathy, remembering how competent and helpful she had always been. They will wonder what made her so disgruntled. Worst of all, they will go to the IRS whistleblower website and learn how laughably easy it is to file a claim. They will rack their brains for questionable schemes they have been exposed to, which the company happens to be loaded up with, to file their own claims before their cube neighbors do. Tax Joe and his co-honchos heard rumors about the rumor and realized Dude was the likely source. George reamed Dude a new one.

After the initial IDRs had been fulfilled and fully processed by the IRS, the second tranche was formulated and then delivered. Whereas the first set had not indicated informed intent, this second set was terrifying. They were at such a level of specificity, so insightfully aggressive, and so numerous while at the same time deeply relevant that Dude felt he had been split wide open. There was nowhere to hide. The IRS knew what they needed and specified those items in unambiguous language. They had deep knowledge of all the business unit complexities and also deep conviction of their case. InsCo obstructed in small ways as if to put up a fight, but these obstructions were trivial. The IRS barreled through like a juggernaut.

Happy days.

Or, my revenge may fall flat. The IRS might decide that they don't have enough staff to pursue this particular issue or that their current portfolio of InsCo tax issues is sufficient. I will get a notice in the mail that the claim has been dropped, and I will never know why.

It is impossible to know which of these scenarios will occur, but I see the claim clearly now. I was right to object so vociferously to the implementation of the treaty ten years ago. Hopefully my actions will prevent this particular theft by the global scumbag-ocracy and instead the money will be returned to the American people to whom it belongs.

We have an obligation to report unethical behavior even if we stand to benefit from doing so. Based on the inherent merits of the claim as I have grown to apprehend them, there is an excellent chance that events are proceeding along the lines of my fantasy above. I nailed them, and I'm glad I did it.

# Chapter 39 - Dad Dead and Brother

∞

When we were children, Dad frequently smoked marijuana in the house. Pot made him relaxed and cheerful, states he otherwise was not usually able to achieve. When we were young teenagers, he offered us puffs on his joints. I turned him down, but Dad and Hunter would sit next to each other in a fragrant cloud, Dad smiling at Hunter, temporarily able to view his son benevolently.

My brother is two years younger than I. I'm not proud of this, but when we were in our teens I thought he was revolting. I remember riding next to him in a car and being disgusted by the pressure of his flesh on mine. He had strong and unpleasant body odor, and he often had a loopy grin and half-lidded eyes. When he had girlfriends in high school, I sensed an aggressive sexuality. This also was disgusting to me. I didn't take an interest in his activities, and he didn't take an interest in mine. Hunter has always been relaxed and nonconfrontational, the very opposite of his hard-charging sisters. What I judged then to be aimlessness and lack of initiative, I now recognize as his cover for isolation and disappointment within our family and his effort to build a confident and easy persona separate from our neglectful parents. I wish things had been different between us back then.

I did him a bit of good when he was seventeen, though, when I challenged him and then beat him soundly at arm wrestling. He had thought he could win because he was a guy. Right before I pounded his pale, unexercised arm down on the table, I taunted him. Pretty much the next day he started running and lifting weights, and he has been fit and strong his whole life since.

He was accepted to a prestigious university for undergraduate studies, which surprised me. I was less surprised when he was kicked out after the first semester under a cloud of bad grades and rumors of drug dealing. After dropping out of college, he worked in Hometown in the restaurant business for many years. He married a cheerful woman, and they made two charming daughters. He smoked pot heavily, well into his forties. His wife and daughters adore him.

Early on Dad helped him buy some investment real estate, and, gradually, over the decades, Dad helped him in other substantial ways, which makes me happy. They went on bike rides and hung out together. Maybe this was a good fit: Hunter's gentle nature next to Dad's peevishness.

When we were both in our late thirties and through our forties, Hunter and I tried to develop a real connection and relationship, which we had never previously had. I visited Hometown a few times, always when my parents were away traveling, and he visited me a couple of times with his family. His daughters are lovely people who were always a delight to be around. He and I spoke on the phone not frequently but regularly. I always called him, and he would invariably say that he had been thinking of me and meaning to call. The conversations centered around his own family and activities, and I accepted this one-sidedness with some disappointment. My brother also worked to develop a relationship with Mom, which he acknowledged he hadn't had growing up. Mom was especially close to Hunter's older girl, who was a Mom mini-me.

When I was around fifty-one and my brother around forty-nine, my father died and left his estate to my brother. Or rather, he left 1 percent of the value to each of the daughters and the rest to Hunter, terms blatantly intended to sow discord. Probably my sisters, like me, received only a small portion of Dad's estate because they had sided with Mom during my parents' divorce and its aftermath. Throughout his life, Dad had devoted his considerable talents to accumulating and retaining assets of value. I wasn't privy to the details of his finances during our decades-long estrangement, but I paid close attention to what my siblings told me about his continued stockpiling of art, real estate, financial investments, and cash. Although I can't be sure, my conservative guess is that his estate had a value in the range of $2 million, which meant Hunter and his family would never worry about money again. I had long felt that the damage done by my parents to Hunter's sweet soul was unconscionable, and I was glad about his family's financial security. A large amount of money can provide contentment when other pieces of your life are in order. Whatever his lack of professional success, with his lovely family my brother does have the basics worked out.

At the same time, I was struggling daily with fatigue, bad sleep, nighttime convulsions that felt like seizures, and dark thoughts. I was haunted by the growing conviction not only that these and other lifelong symptoms were the result of my parent's negligence, but also that my parents had hidden this truth from me to save themselves shame. They had thereby denied me the knowledge that would otherwise have enabled me to manage my illness and prevent my ultimate disability. In my last conversation with Hunter, he told me the results of Dad's will, and I pleaded with him to share more of the estate with the three daughters. I said that this man had done enormous damage to all of us, that the terms of the will were deliberately destructive to the family, and that Hunter had the means to partially redress a long-term injustice. He could lay the groundwork for reconciliation among the siblings in the future. I said that considering the likely size of the estate, $100,000 for each of the daughters was the right amount. Hunter insisted he would honor Dad's intent and then said, in these words, "I'm going to do exactly what I want."

This is what a child says about a candy bar, not what a grown man says to his sister about their ghastly family history. The "fuck you, I'm keeping it all" philosophy was more typical of my father than what I remembered of Hunter. They had spent a lot of time together in recent years. Maybe softheaded Hunter in middle age began to finally identify with Dad and was channeling Dad to justify his own status as primary heir. I ended the call in disgust.

I see now that my reaction wasn't about the money, which I would have regarded as tainted. Instead, I was deeply hurt that my brother did not care about my suffering. Perhaps he hadn't listened when I told him how ill I was, or perhaps his history of drug use made him habitually forget much of what he was told. I had had considerable career and job instability as I repeatedly became ill in different workspaces and left jobs abruptly. Even though I had some savings and my house was paid for, I had feelings of financial insecurity on top of deep health insecurity. For several days, I was angry and upset. My brother's unwillingness to fully inform himself of my circumstances was a shriek in my face that he didn't care about me. I thought of how I had always called him and listened to him *ad tedium* and how I had suppressed evidence of his limited scope. I was unable to forgive him. We children all competed for Dad's love and approval, and my brother was finally receiving a large expression of both. This zero-sum transfer was especially sweet for Hunter because it happened at the expense of his highly educated and professionally accomplished sisters. I was bitterly disappointed that he was not able to rise above this childish longing and do what I thought was the right thing.

When Hunter was a child, there was a lightness about him and a pure enjoyment of life, which I am sure he still has. But my parents didn't take an interest in his development, and he was left to make his own way. I think when he was so badly beaten by Dad as a boy and young teen that he lost his will to accomplish things in the wider world. In later years when the two of them became close, probably Dad was trying to compensate for the early damage he had done.

Now, a few years after this call with Hunter, I see things differently. My rush to find him wanting means I hadn't developed empathy, maybe because we never were simpatico—or maybe because a small and guilty part of me still judged him aimless and another small and even more guilty part of me still found him revolting. I was being dishonest during those phone calls, listening to him blab on about his life while thinking I was doing him a favor. I did have feelings for him, but I also knew that I hadn't found a way to build a connection with him that had a true basis. It was Hunter who put up with Dad and loved him after the rest of the family fell away. It wasn't a surprise that Dad's will was malicious. I don't have a claim on Hunter's money.

∾

Dad had mild dementia in his last years. In fact, the Bedbug told me that Dad's dementia was the primary reason Mom divorced him. This apparent—not actual—causality reveals more about the Bedbug's cold heart than it does about the final deterioration of my parents' relationship.

Dad was extremely vain and body conscious. He frequently asked us if his ass looked flat in his jeans, to which we were supposed to say of course not, and he always wanted to be thinner, which he equated with increased beauty. In his later years he had a tendency to eat lightly, and I'm sure with the onset of his dementia he didn't have common sense about proper nutrition for himself. I didn't see him for thirty years. Near the end of his life, my siblings all told me that he was tiny, like a bird. But despite his anorexia, if rich food were put in front of him that he hadn't had to prepare and that he wasn't paying for, he would wolf it down.

When Dad was around eighty and after Mom divorced him, Hunter moved him into a house near Hunter's family. Dad paid Hunter a few thousand dollars a month to help him with practical matters. I urged Hunter to get Dad's memory loss and cognitive impairment properly tested and diagnosed, but to my knowledge this never happened. Evidently his personality mellowed. He shuffle-jogged daily around a nearby park and had lunch once a week with cronies from his bicycle racing age bracket. Nasty man finally has some measure of peace and companionship near his family.

But here's the rub. When Hunter called me to tell me that Dad had died, it wasn't clear what killed him. There was a collapse, and then a fairly short hospitalization with peeing and pooping while comatose, and then he was dead. I quizzed Hunter about the cause of death, and he told me no one knew. We conjectured that the many sporting, driving, and home-renovation head traumas had caused the dementia, but the final physical decline seemed mysterious and precipitous. Then, remembering how thin Dad had been, I suggested nutritional deficiencies had contributed to his rapid deterioration. My brother responded, no lie: "Yeah, probably. You can't really live on Cheez-Its and oatmeal." So here is the lesson: if you create a dope-addled son, whom you never fed properly when he was a child and who is going to inherit your largish estate, you had best not put that son in charge of your meals.

Over the years my father had been so ill-natured to his other local adult family, meaning Amy, Mom, and Hunter's wife, that none of them were going to bring him food either. How much trouble would it have been to stop by daily with takeout, meaning a cheeseburger, some sweet-and-sour pork, or a meatloaf blue plate special? Just like a baby bird, he would have gratefully inhaled whatever hot food was set in front of him. Surely there is a service that delivers a large meal daily in exchange for a credit card number. No one wanted him to live longer, so they all colluded in accepting his tiny body and haunted, hungry eyes.

Hunter was vague about a funeral service, and I suspected he couldn't be bothered. Our parents hadn't taught us either the necessity or the execution skills for such social conventions anyway. I might have liked to attend a ceremony, to make sure Dad was dead, but traveling isn't possible for me.

A year after Dad died I got a check for $5,000, representing my 1 percent share. Hunter explained in the accompanying letter that the estate was valued at half a million dollars. No way was Dad worth so relatively little after a lifetime of Scrooge-like miserliness and Midas-like real estate and art investments, even after divorce bifurcation. Estate taxes don't kick in until much higher levels of valuation, so the only motivation my brother could have for such an undervaluation was to send his three sisters as little as possible for their 1 percent share. Did he think we were stupid? This evidence of disregard and see-through perfidy was another blow.

Who was my brother, and who was I to him? We tried to make something out of a few old memories and what we saw in the other of well-intentioned interest, but our affection was not sufficient in the end. With respect to my family, I'd had a clean sweep. They were all gone.

# Chapter 40 - Who I Am Now

All my life I've had a sense of foreboding. I knew something was wrong with me. This was partly because my parents hadn't found kindness and instead blamed me for their own hidden burdens, but also because I couldn't trust my levels of energy or the vagaries of my mental state. I did my best to shore up resources against the unidentified weakness within myself. I made good grades, worked hard in jobs, saved money, worked with Husband to renovate our purchased houses, kept myself fit, was gracious to neighbors, paid off mortgages as soon as possible, and ate healthy foods. There was no room to be careless or unkind, take drugs, get drunk, goof off at work, accumulate consumer debt, buy expensive clothing, or beget children.

As I suffered unexplained health setbacks that caused me repeatedly to lose jobs and friends, I sensed further catastrophe coming but didn't know what form it would take. I continued to do the best work I could at my jobs and continued to save money, basically more of the same according to the common-sense rules of our society. Catastrophe did come. During a few exceptionally terrible years, I lost my health, my job, my ability to work for money, the vestiges of my family, and my mobility in the world. I was forced to move away from the city where I had lived for thirty-five years and the community connections I had built during that time. I lost interest in hobbies, and I lost vast swaths of memory.

My lifelong caution bailed me out when the shit hit the fan. Because of my profile and history, I was able to claw back my job and keep it for a few more crucial years, borrow money to buy the new house without relying on cash from the old one, use our experience renovating houses to make the new one nontoxic and therefore safe, and later be a credible reporter when applying for social security disability benefits. I survived the life cataclysm that had been looming, against which I had, even at ages eleven and twelve, hoarded my babysitting earnings and tried to please my teachers.

My brain, trained to expect misfortune, cannot now enjoy an easy contentment. Decades of strategizing and striving have given me a habit of mental fermentation. Since losing my job, I have written applications for two utility patents and have prosecuted these patents without a lawyer. I have gotten a trademark, established two Etsy shops, run Kickstarter campaigns, continued with home renovations, set up a sculpture workshop, and applied for numerous artist fellowships. I'm taking steps to revive my workers' compensation case. I have set ambitious landscaping plans in motion and learned how to knit socks on a machine and how to sew panties. For the last county fair, I made submissions in twelve different home arts categories and received nine first-place ribbons and two second-place ribbons. But what is the point? Throughout this bubbling of current activity, I am burdened with sadness and regrets over my past life and who I am now.

When I was a child, I loved small children, cats, and dogs, and now I don't even like them. I was kind to others by default, and now I'm just not. I am quick to see flaws in people and inclined to see myself as better than others, which is ironic considering how much neuro-damage I have had. When I see a person my age with a limp I want to yell, "Do your yoga!" and when I see a fat person, "Eat . . . less . . . cake!" I blame others for misfortunes I believe they could have prevented, but how can I expect them to be as careful as I was forced to be?

I am burdened that when I was a child, I let the wrong people into my heart. I was gutted, and for decades afterward I scrambled to recover balance and wholeness. Like an imprinted duckling, I clung to my family, and, when they fell away, my heart was empty and still is. I still sometimes say to myself that I don't want new people; I want *those* people.

It is time to reboot my life. My job now is to fully accept that one of the key disadvantages of being a child is that you are an automatic dumbshit. I have to forgive myself for these ancient decisions as well as for the person I have become.

On the upside, I am not ill most days because my new life mechanics are effective. I have a simple unassuming wardrobe that is machine-washed only. Wardrobe staples, like long-sleeved T-shirts and woven summer tops, I sew myself from organic fabrics. Because personal care products make me sick, my standards for hygiene and grooming are those of a Victorian scullery maid. Because I distrust the chemicals in toothpaste, I have a system of dental care that involves a lot of scrubbing and crevice excavation with wooden sticks, and my dentist loves me for my gums. Unfortunately, I'm still fecund at age fifty-five, meaning menstruating, but I use washable cloth pads instead of toxic tampons or fragranced disposable pads. I sew my own tissues from organic muslin and cut my own hair in a "good-enough" layered bob. I have discovered that regularly eating fermented vegetables has changed my biome such that my armpit BO is negligible for many days after a bath. Also, when I drop my dirt, there is almost no smell. I walk to our primary grocery store with a cart pulled by one hand and a respirator held in the other against car and truck exhaust. One of the best decisions Husband and I ever made was his vasectomy many years ago, so we have a chemical-free intimate life. I use various lawn-minimizing landscaping techniques to reduce mowing, air-dry our laundry, and strip the snail mail down to bare bones while wearing a respirator before bringing any of it into the house. I don't go places, generally.

I see my story clearly. In the past I let things happen to me because I accepted relationships at face value. I was wrong about how my family members felt toward me. During my time in the corporate world, I was wrong about the true level of regard that colleagues and supervisors had for me. I was wrong about the true nature of consumer products, building materials, and many other chemical substances that fill our world. I was wrong about the capacity of our societal infrastructure, meaning regulators, doctors, and producers of the items in our workspaces and homes, to protect us from harm. In all of these cases, the truth was the direct opposite of what I was told.

Harrowing experiences can crush us, but they can also give us wisdom unattainable by other means. I must now use my expensive wisdom to retrain my brain, that sad and much abused organ, and reinvent myself for the next fifty years of my life.

# Chapter 41 - Who Was My Mother?

∞

Husband and I run a woodstove in our kitchen in the winter-time, and we use the old coal-storage room in the basement for storing cordwood. Like the rest of our basement, it has an eight-foot ceiling and a concrete floor, is dry, and has walls that are brick on top of fieldstone. There is one small window to the driveway, which we use as a wood chute when we have cordwood delivered, and a metal fire door that has the weight and construction of a ship's boiler room door. I love stacking wood, splitting large pieces, and sorting kindling in this room. The room is large, about ten feet by twenty. We had the bricks repointed, the room cleaned up, electricity run to it, and a couple of light fixtures put in. It is underneath a porch and has gaps here and there to the outside. Although it is mostly underground, because of these gaps it doesn't benefit from geothermal warming as much as the rest of the basement and can get quite cold. For the first couple of years I felt happiness and mild awe whenever I entered this room, like some people do in a cathedral.

There is evidence of chipmunk activity, like stores of chokecherry pits and a small doorway, a smooth hole between two foundation stones underneath which there is sometimes new dirt. If I inadvertently disturb one of the chipmunk's caches as I work through a woodpile, the next day the cache has been cleaned up and moved. So far this winter I have been leaving a treat every night in a little dish—an olive pit, an overcooked chestnut, a split walnut. Every morning the offering is gone, and I am thrilled to once again achieve communication across a great distance.

A few days ago, I went to retrieve wood and disturbed a small colony of regular ants who had settled for the winter between two stacked pieces. There were about fifty of them and some clusters of eggs on a flat, clean section of split wood, a little helter-skelter by the time I noticed them. Perhaps this was only a portion of the colony, and the rest was tucked somewhere else. Most were still, but some moved slowly in the cold dark air. Our house is free of creatures except for bats, a large population of spiders, and the occasional super-speedy insectivore centipede, and I don't regard any of these as vermin. Ants of this size won't harm our house and are not a chronic problem. I set the piece of wood aside, keeping it level, planning to put it in a sheltered place outside when a forecasted snowstorm had come and gone. The next day, I checked the ants. They had organized themselves into stringy clumps on top of and completely covering the egg clusters. Even partially dormant and with their colony disturbed, totally exposed to any danger, they had one collective priority: protect the children.

This is where I struggle. If a few clumps of tiny and frozen ants can agree on the most important thing and act immediately based on this priority, why was my mother, a basically kindhearted and reasonable person, not able to summon even a tiny bit of concern for my well-being? How could she have stood by silently when I became so ill with what I told other family members was chemical sensitivities while I tried desperately to figure out the underlying cause and how to manage the illness? Why do I still not know her?

She was a normal person of average intelligence and looks. She married a charismatic and extremely handsome man whose core was deeply damaged. Even as she identified my father's deficiencies during their early years together, she was unwilling to leave the marriage. This was because of her fear of abandonment, both from her own father's death when she was a small child and from her mother's consequent emotional withdrawal. My mother also kept her marriage because she wanted to consider herself more successful than her two sisters, each of whom happened to have had an early failed marriage.

When my parents were first married, the basic largesse of their world and their own attributes and placement within that world predicted a fairly contented life together. Two events intervened, both borne of arrogance and bad luck. First, together, through negligence, they accidentally and irrevocably injured the lifelong health of one of their children, which only became fully apparent to them drip-style over a period of several years. Second, my father indulged in secret sexual- and admiration-based meditations about one of their children. It was the same child in both cases, namely me. For my mother, guilt over the early injury and cover-up, jealousy, and self-hatred from these seedy impulses bred an uncontrollable antipathy toward me.

The relaxed social mores of the time and of their university community and my father's tendency toward rage when challenged prevented other family members, friends, or social services from interfering in the family's affairs. Also, my father created a mythology that our family was better than any other family, and this fascist religion stopped family members from telling outsiders what happened in our home. The two of them were able to feed and clothe their children badly and he was able to beat them while both continued to be seen as worthy members of society, middle-class professionals, and even upstanding intellectuals. My mother didn't insist on proper clothes, nutrition, medical care, or life guidance for the three youngest children because her ethical core was eroded by living with my father and also because she was lazy. My father thought his children's needs made unreasonable demands on his hoarded assets, and he didn't encourage his children's natural gifts because these gifts were threats to his own self-worth.

What a fucking disaster.

After the lawsuit, I persisted in attributing kindly intentions to my mother. I imagined that she missed me and that my absence weighed upon her daily, that she thought of me and felt an eroding wave when she woke up in the middle of the night. I was sure she wanted me to be healthy and happy in my marriage and at my jobs.

Now I struggle mightily toward an alternative evidence- and reality-based version of my mother's view of me. I see that my presence as a young child was a nagging burden, a reminder of a horrific episode of negligence and resulting neurological injury when I was a baby. Later, there were times when I was either ill or unusually withdrawn for periods of a year or more that were especially painful for her. She hoped to make me smaller and weaker and that my presence in her life would wither. She did not look at me closely to assess my condition or offer advice. She savored news of my life's disruptions because she could interpret these disruptions as signs that I was the deficient person, not her. Then, at last, a breach meant that contact was infrequent and later nonexistent. She felt light, free to travel with her favorite children and enjoy her grandchildren, free to renew her physical relationship with Dad, free to develop hobbies and become super fit. The ongoing reminder of that distant horrific event was finally gone.

If I am to view my past life with clarity and build a new life, I must repudiate romantic garbage based on magical thinking. With extreme discipline and even brutality, I must see that my mother has nothing for me. I don't know her because she never wanted me to.

If my parents had acknowledged the truth of the cause of my early illness to themselves and to others, they probably would have become careful and humble people. Social shame can be cleansing, and people can find redemption through atonement. My father would not have become an ill-tempered and preening hoarder of cash, toys, and solo experiences, and my mother wouldn't have sat on the steps of the porch with her friends, drinking a beer while six months pregnant. My illness could have been managed, and I would not have been crippled.

I have remembered, and now I understand. I want to put this sad past behind me, and for this I must stop looking backward. I want to live out the rest of my life in a space that doesn't make me ill, and for this I must stay home. Chocolate, religion, a little bit of wine, a picture book, some marijuana, family, a nice perfume, a yoga class—all the classic pick-me-ups are unavailable to me. What will it be instead? Home-based creative activities, online movies and education, making healthful meals with Sweetie-pie, and sitting in the garden. A year ago I thought it would require heavy lifting and luck to build a life from these meager components. Now I have them all in play, and, except for leftover sadness, it's just fine.

Do I get in the girls, meaning the gargantuan hens, so that their flat-lining reptilian brains can calm my own fevered wrinkle-mush? And should Husband and I get a toxi-box just so we can go out into the countryside once a month, even if we need to wear respirators to sit inside the toxi-box? Am I confusing acquisition with accomplishment? Ordering up five female chicks and a car is not the same as having the internal fortitude to find contentment in every moment that I am not chem-crapped. But maybe I have already demonstrated enough internal fortitude in my life.

# Chapter 42 - The Naked Fucker

As I stay home and my health improves, more memories are returning. I learned how to read when I was three. When I was six, I had a scavenged pet—a huge albino cockroach that I kept in a large matchbox. I took this pet to school and let it run up my arm and over my body.

My aunt Rose, the profoundly unlucky woman who married Dad's troubled brother, recently told me about a visit my family made to hers when I was around ten years old. She saw Dad pull me onto his lap and do something that gave her dread. She felt helpless at the time, and the memory haunted her. She wouldn't tell me what happened, only that the contact was sexual and that I wanted to get away from him.

With respect to how a fecund and wrong-minded man thinks about women, there is a scale that runs from piglet, through swine, to sexual predator. I try to assess my father's position on this scale, but when I remember the things he said and did, I cannot think clearly because the events are too close to me and I see them through a child's eyes. I need distance.

In the late 1970s, my father published some autobiographical fiction describing the academic milieu of that time. Before the book was published and when it was in draft form, I got a dollar from him for each typo I found, but I haven't read the book in forty years. Modern technology has put all of the world's knowledge at our fingertips, so via the interweb and shipped for free, I recently ordered up a like-new hardcopy of this tawdry tome for $5. I hoped this version of his voice would help me discern his inner life.

My father the narrator has a large vocabulary and uses colorful and evocative language. He is thoughtful, observant, and occasionally genuinely funny, but at the same time he is self-aggrandizing and therefore cannot be trusted. The way he writes about women must have been distressing to my mother and her feminist friends at the time, and it makes my skin crawl today. The book isn't pornographic, but there are frequent appreciative references to female body parts as well as to penises. It has the exploitative flair of pornography. He writes about walking across campus staring at "lolling bosoms" and hoping to catch a glimpse of "beaver." I know it was the 1970s, but really—"beaver"!? My father comes across as a self-satisfied and hopeful voyeur, an entitled snob, a swaggering Norman Mailer–esque partial person continually assessing the sexual availability and offerings of others. He is all about the looking and the judging. If you don't appear as though you might "trick," you don't rate. After reading in his book a little while, I feel his selfish presence again. I want that paper artifact out of my house and then a bath.

I remember: When I went home for Christmas at age seventeen during freshman year, Mom and Dad picked me up at the airport. Dad hugged me for way too long and then asked me if my body was still supple. It was just plain weird. While it was happening, I noticed Mom observing with an assessing tight-lipped expression on her face. Later that day I told her that I was uncomfortable with the hug and strongly sensed that she, grim of heart, knew immediately what I was talking about. If I hadn't mentioned the long weird hug, she would have been able to continue sort of pimping me out, meaning semi-colluding in Dad's sexual impulses to keep him contented. She figured I would leave their home and be back at school soon enough. I don't mean full-scale rape. I mean one-sided flirting, looking at my body, lots of sitting quietly and thinking about my body, and more of his signature penis reveals.

Kirsten had also come home from college, so all six of us were together. Christmas morning, Dad told us children that he and Mom were unable to handle being in the house with us. Probably he referred to that old standby, family turbulence. They got in the car, drove off, and stayed away until late that evening. We children were mystified. We had not behaved badly, and yet we were blamed for some evil intent that they discerned but we could not. There was never more of an explanation for their departure, and the family never had a Christmas dinner or communal gift-opening that year. We children took the turkey out of the oven at some point and tore pieces off of it, and now I imagine that Mom and Dad took themselves to a lovely meal at a nice local hotel and then went for a drive in the country and maybe a movie in the late afternoon. Not that they were happy, but they made the best of it. The issue was that Mom couldn't stand looking at me. She forced Dad to make excuses for the two of them to get them both away from me for the day that we otherwise would have spent together as a family.

When they brought me back to the airport a couple of days later, Mom watched closely as Dad mechanically gave me a short embrace. At that moment, I saw that the two of them had a long-term understanding about his feelings for me. I promptly suppressed that knowledge.

I used to read a lot; really, all the time. Now when I want to read, my mind races ahead and I have trouble concentrating.

Probably because of neurological damage, I have trouble absorbing and retaining new information. I've lost vocabulary. But there is a deeper reason for my disinterest in the written word: there are few people whose voices I trust. I have been badly damaged by so many huge lies, lies that served the purposes of other people, that now I'm not interested in what other people have to say. So little has the ring of truth. One week coffee is bad for you, and the next it contains the keys to vanquishing all disease. One year Christopher Columbus was a hero, and twenty years later he was a destructive man. When I was a teenager, beauty products and new clothes were worthwhile objects of pursuit, and now they make me ill and contribute to environmental destruction. I know for a fact that cars are toxic boxes, yet this is nowhere in the collective consciousness. Where are the most important truths? I've come to believe they are in reality-based, science-based clarity of thought and extreme caution. Avoid giving yourself to people who are not generous and kindhearted. Lay off the novels and sitcoms, and don't believe 70 percent of what you read in the news. Stay home as much as you practically can.

The last time that Dad and I were around each other much was when I was fifteen. He loomed large in my mind well into my thirties because I was struggling. I wasn't able to stop hoping that he would help me or show me kindness, but he wasn't an actual presence in my life during those years. What was he like when I was fifteen? He was rude and dismissive to me while continually claiming that I was being rude and mean to him, which I wasn't, and he repeatedly showed me his penis—yuck. It is easy to dismiss him as a selfish jerk, but the peevishness and, clearly seen, sexual assault are truth signifiers. If I bear down, I can learn something.

Like Mom, Dad was a broken person, unable to either process or accommodate the contradictions he felt when he looked at me. He saw that I was accomplished in school, responsible at chores, and creative at making things, but also that I regularly became ill and depressed for months or even years at a time. He saw that I was lovely and full of grace, but he also sensed my shapeliness and fragrance during years when he wasn't having all the sex he wanted from other sources. He saw that I was cheerful, kindhearted, and generous, all of which reminded him that he was not. He saw my curiosity about the world and my deep optimism and resilience, and he knew that my hidden health damage made this optimism unjustified because my life was a bad lookout. He made me, but because he also broke me, I ruined his wife, his marriage, his tranquility, and his belief in his own basic goodness and the goodness of the world. So he and Mom treated me badly, which made them feel even worse.

I remember how they looked at me when they made me move out of their house when I was fifteen; when they met my friends at my college graduation; when they were across the conference table from me at the legal deposition. Reflected in their eyes is what they saw—a rogue turd bolus, swirling around and around and around and refusing to go down. If it's true that I'm locked in a decades-long death match with these people, I'm the one who is going to win. One down, one to go.

The artist Goya created a dark painting that he never titled but that was posthumously and mistakenly named by others *Saturn Devouring His Son*. The image shows a giant unclothed crouching man, eyes rolling in his head, holding upright with both hands a much smaller body. He has already eaten the head and is starting on the shoulders, like you would an ice cream cone. The small partial body, seen from the back, is obviously that of a woman, not a man, as it has a woman's rounded buttocks, shapely legs, and soft shoulders. Here is a truth: that crazed naked fucker was my father, and I am the one he wanted to consume and destroy. Here is a truth: my mother is pitiful and chose her husband badly, but she wasn't an innocent and she did me a great deal of damage. Here is another truth: I worked for fifteen years for an ethically bereft company that uses unconscionable devices to evade taxes. And here is the biggest truth: Because there is no one minding the shop, we are surrounded by toxic substances that are damaging our health and the health of our loved ones. We cannot believe what we are told about the consumer goods around us but must view them with extreme clarity of mind and avoid, avoid, avoid.

# Chapter 43 - The Plumbers

This story is not of the life I wanted. My initial chemical injury, my parents' denial of it, and the pervasiveness of fragrances and toxins around me circumscribed the scope of my life. Within my birth family and at InsCo, tax exploitation and sexual bias or assault—those hand-in-hand signifiers of corrupted patriarchy—further constrained me. I grew up on the false religion of self-determination and remained ignorant of the hidden factors undermining my careful choices and hard work. Gentle reader, hidden factors are at work in your world also. Your health and the health of your loved ones are being undermined by your material infrastructure without your knowledge. Environmental destruction and toxic products are manifestations of the lies and heedless grabbing of neoliberalism and also the ultimate expression of its failure.

Sometimes people achieve one great thing, and that is enough. Think about the folks who wrote that amazing song, "Who Let the Dogs Out?" Actually, only that one line in that song. They should sit the fuck down, having justified their existence by the immeasurable happiness they brought to the world through a single accomplishment. When I was young,

I thought I was destined for great things, and for years I felt disappointed at my own lack of achievement. But the funds of resilience, determination, good faith, and creativity that I was born with might have had no higher purpose than enabling me to survive. For me, that single achievement is sufficient. I, too, can stop striving and sit the fuck down.

If I look back at my younger self, I see the greatest distance across which I would like to communicate. I want to give this adorable child the gift of important information, but what can I say? The deck is stacked against you. Your parents truly suck. Your life will be one of unusual bad luck and will not be anything like you anticipate. What possible advice or consolation could alleviate the shitstorm that was going to surround me for decades? The only information I could have made good use of was what my parents devoted themselves to concealing. Hey, you—you are horrifically ill, orphaned, and surrounded by creeps, and you won't know it for another forty crappy years. Best not to think about it.

Six years ago I was ill, and few objects around me were safe. Now by living a restricted life, I get acceptable levels of sleep and feel some wellness most of the time. After several months during which I said to myself almost daily that I needed some good news, my application for social security disability was approved. The money will provide long-term financial security, and this official validation of my condition will make it easier for me to get understanding and support during future medical visits. Ever a worrier and planner, I can now rest easier concerning the basic mechanics of my future.

I have had horrific trauma and loss, but I feel sure the basic life components I have assembled can make me somewhat cheerful in the future. My mind is not rotten anymore, so my "fake it till you make it" checklist has gradually transitioned to a cheering menu of gentle domestic blisses and pleasurable options—yay!

Does it count as a loss, if it was never yours in the first place? I realize now that all I have lost was never really mine. I thought I could move around normally in the world, travel, drive a car, make and keep friends. But even before I became so ill at age forty-eight, I often felt vague discomfort and slight fatigue after shopping or eating in a restaurant. I slept badly when I traveled and felt ill at ease and disconnected driving a car. It was hard for me to keep friends, and I rarely felt happy at parties or other social gatherings. I thought I was middle-class, first as a computer professional and later as an accountant, but I was just trying to claw back a career that kept slipping away from me, again and again, until it was well and truly gone.

The most wrenching loss was my family. Sometimes I still feel heartache and a soul-splintering longing for these people. I cherished a future with each of them, but I had never possessed their love and regard. What I had instead were relationships that were fatally broken from the start, years of longing and hurt, a load of old shit. My brother and Aunt Cynthia, not so much, but when I now consider my dead father, my sisters, my mother, I see festering turds.

In Franklin County, Massachusetts, workmen are pleasant, intelligent, and responsive. Passing by two bearded older white guys in plaid shirts near the post office, I overhear them discussing berry gardens, not the Boston Bruins. What a relief. Our house has nine bedrooms and six bathrooms and was in some disrepair when we bought it, so it has required a great deal of attention by contractors. Husband and I have been happy with the work done by each of the trades—except for plumbing. Plumbers around here are overpriced and unreliable divas. Why? Because they perform the demanding and vitally important work of getting the shit away from the house. Compared to the exigency of successfully routing human dirt down the waste pipes and off the property, exploding tubes of asbestos and sagging porches are inconsequential. These guys know their own worth.

We should all learn how to do a bit of basic plumbing. All of us should be able to locate and eliminate a stinky pucky that we have the misfortune to come into contact with in our domain. As years pass and I just stay home, my health will continue to improve and my mind will clear. Like others in my matriarchal line, I will live a long time. With sweet words and fistfuls of cash, I will persuade a local plumber to fix the leaky faucets and get the far-flung bathrooms working again. I will rest in contentment and with a measure of nobility upon these distant thrones and unburden myself in happy solitude. With a clear memory, I will vigilantly avoid contact with my family, the festerings. With patience and an unapologetic savoring of vengeance, as I receive second-hand reports of deteriorating health and death after death, I will be unburdened, lightened. It is the entrails that are the true source of human emotional and spiritual sufficiency, and my empty and healthy bowel will beget a healed and pure white soul.

# Afterword

$\infty$

It takes a while for a book to be published so there has been news since I wrote the final chapter of this memoir. I googled my childhood sweetheart, Richard. He became a math teacher as he always said he would, but he is divorced and has been arrested twice: once for embezzling money from a high school fund for students, and the second time for shoplifting steaks from a grocery store. I can't recognize him in the puffy-faced mugshots and feel saddened and unsettled. Then I remember that I dumped him because he was bossy and am heartened by this evidence of my own common sense.

I'd forgotten his last name but my mother's therapist, Bruce, pops right up when I google "Bruce therapist Hometown." Bruce died of gastric cancer many years ago when he was in his sixties. I'm glad he is dead only because this frees me from fantasizing about shaking him down for a confession. The photos and obituary creep me out a little bit.

I get a Christmas newsletter from my mother's younger sister, Gloria, and learn that Aunt Cynthia the Bedbug has rapidly progressing Alzheimer's. She has moved out of New York City and into Mom's house in Hometown so that Mom can take care of her. I am not surprised by my mother's generosity and fortitude. Husband and I had gently teased Cynthia about padding to the door of her apartment first thing every morning, rubbing the sleep out of her eyes with the knuckles of one hand while reaching down for the folded daily *New York Times* with the other. I remember how she used to moisten her fingers to separate the pages and think surely there is a link between her current neurological deterioration and all those decades of licking printer's ink for an hour every day.

Our current political climate has provided more context for my family members. I suspect that my mother and Kirsten were Obama voters and then rabid Hillary supporters and that Amy followed their lead. Dad couldn't be bothered to vote and, ugh, Hunter owns a MAGA hat and considers himself a Trump supporter although he isn't actually registered to vote.

I gird my "lions" and place a call to the woman coordinating my IRS whistleblower's claim. We both acknowledge that she is prohibited from telling me anything other than whether or not the claim is still active. It is. This excellent news means that after just about three years the IRS has dug in because they are optimistic of success. I am filled with joy for several days knowing how much trouble, worry, and expense I have caused InsCo. Also, maybe I will be rich, which will give me and Husband a buffer against life's slings and arrows.

These days I don't go out much at all, and my sleep is good almost every night. Husband and I are happy from day to day. One recent day, I woke up and realized that the shadow of trauma and loss that was so heavy a year ago that I thought it would always be with me, was gone. I lay in bed in the dark, poking here and there at the past events that used to be guaranteed triggers for sadness and regret and felt nothing. All of those terrible things happened to the me of then, not the me of now.

The remaining members of my family, those ridiculous specimens, no longer have any pull on me. My inner resilience must
be off the charts. I'm the one they should study! For decades, I
was searching for what was important in life and unable to find
it because my obliviousness of my own condition made me blind
to the workings of the world. This memoir has helped me see
the truth and also made me think I can be a writer. I have found
my voice, I like the sound of it, and I've started to set my sights
higher than simple survival.

I see more and more articles about studies that link
fragrances and other pervasive, unregulated chemicals to neurological damage specifically, although so far the authors of
these studies have been seemingly afraid of fully presenting the
underlying truths. My local librarians are lovely and gracious,
and I feel terrible that the building where they spend their days
smells like crappy carpeting and other cheap and toxic building
components. I feel the same for the workers at the local Home
Depot and the tellers at my bank. I wish there was some way
I could tell them what I know. If I tried I would just seem like
a deranged person, with my bad clothes and un-made-up face,
searching for the right words and failing. I want to raise my voice
against this threat, but, at the same time, I know that people
ignore inconvenient truths until the dangers are too apparent to
be denied. Just like everyone knew that cigarettes caused health
damage, everyone knows that the chemicals around us are injur-
ing our brains, but we don't yet have the language and scientific
framework to hang our hats on it. We need to stop pretending
that we don't know these chemicals are seriously messing us up,
and we need to start taking direct action to avoid them. If we as
consumers stop spending money on toxic garbage and if we as
citizens push for better decisions regarding the products used to
build, furnish, and clean our public spaces, then the scientists,

doctors, politicians, and manufacturers will follow our lead. In this way, we can force them to help us have less toxic air, water, food, consumer products, building materials, and cars. We *must* open our eyes to this most important truth about our world.

# Appendix - Resources and Basic Protocols

As I discussed in Chapter 1, my malady is not an allergy, but is instead an intolerance triggered by a single initiating chemical exposure when I was a baby. Dr. Claudia Miller coined the term toxicant-induced loss of tolerance (TILT), and her website (www.tiltresearch.org) is the best technical resource for sufferers from TILT. Dr. Miller makes the connection between the rise of modern chemical compounds derived from oil, coal, or gas and the emergence of a new disease process in which susceptible individuals show disproportionate symptoms from substances that they previously were able to tolerate. The central premise of my book is that I and others who suffer from TILT are the canaries in the coal mine and that the everyday fragrances and other chemicals that have such extreme effects on us aren't healthy for anyone. In this appendix, I have built on the suggestions at the end of Chapter 7 but have kept my advice high-level. My website (www.pookiesekmet.com) contains additional guidance and examples. For consumer product recommendations and relevant news and analysis, I recommend the Environmental

Working Group website (www.ewg.org), Breast Cancer Prevention Partners (www.BCPP.org), and other similar online resources. Green Building Supply (www.greenbuildingsupply.com) is also a great resource.

The best overall approaches to reducing the amount of toxic stuff entering your life are first, limiting consumption, and second, getting as much use as you can out of items you already own that you have determined to be safe. We are living through a dark time regarding the contamination of our environments by untested, unregulated, or known toxic substances.

## BODY

### *Nourish the body*

Be careful about the sourcing of your food. Work toward cooking simple meals from scratch from organic ingredients that have not been exposed to packaging that might contaminate them. Try not to purchase items from any region that has a reputation for food scandals or insufficient oversight of food production, even if these items are labeled "organic." Husband and I trust our local farmers who have chemical-free farms but can't afford organic certification, we trust organic food from California and other US states, but we do not trust organic food from China.

Our society is in active denial of the full weight of the side effects of many medications. I know I'm oversimplifying, but here goes: birth control pills cause depression, and antidepressants destroy your libido. Also, statins cause constipation, and steroids destroy your cartilage. In recent news items, perpetrators of socially outrageous acts, like the young American man who smeared himself with his own excrement and then walked naked through an airport, have blamed their behavior on their medications. These stories may be funny, but let's not ignore the fact that these medications have the potential to seriously mess us up. I believe that environmental contamination is the root cause for many chronic medical conditions. If you are able to reduce your exposure to chemical toxins, you will be less likely to need long-term medications. Avoid those that are discretionary, like birth control pills.

## *Clean the body*

My own approach to personal hygiene is minimalist—maybe some of these solutions will work for you. I have been able to reduce my armpit body odor by regularly eating raw fermented vegetables, either homemade or store-bought. My overall body biome is improved and balanced, and in this way my armpit biome has become less stinksome. I have also found that dabbing the juice from the jar of vegetables on the armpits works to reduce stink. I have a single moisturizer that I use on my face and the rest of my body. I make it myself from sweet almond oil, beeswax, witch hazel, borax, and vitamin E. The recipe is on my website.

I discovered a lovely age-defying trick recently. As part of my daily exercise routine, I massage my scalp, face, and neck, which feels fantastic. After a few months of this, I discovered that the fine lines on my face and neck were disappearing. I realized that as I alternated scratching my scalp and rubbing my face, the normal healthy oils on my scalp from not washing my hair daily were acting as an amazing anti-wrinkle agent.

I have stopped using toothpaste. Along with it giving me all of the usual symptoms of toxic exposure, regular commercial toothpaste makes me generate a great deal of thick mucus for many hours after brushing. Sometimes this mucus becomes stinky and foul-tasting, which is disgusting. I do a scrubbing and crevice excavation just about every day with wooden sticks while I'm watching a movie or listening to a book on tape. I use Perio-Aid brand toothpick holders, by Marquis Dental Mfg. Co., or a similar stick holder that I fashioned from the handle of an old toothbrush to hold little wooden wedges or plain birch toothpicks.

After I scrub with a wooden stick, I douche my nasal passages and rinse my mouth with weak saltwater and then give my mouth and tongue a little brushing with the salt water, using a toothbrush. I'm experimenting with this still, but I've come to believe that the mouth's natural biome will keep itself sweet if you go easy on it. Whereas, if you flood it with antibacterial products, the healthy biome will die off, too. Then there is a bacterial bloom when the broad-based antibacterial components wear off, and this stinky explosion of uncontrolled harmful bacteria makes you reach for the antibacterial toothpaste or mouthwash again. If you keep your stomach healthy and your gums and sinuses free of infection, these additional sources of potential stink are also eliminated.

The vaginal membrane is more absorptive of medicine and other materials than external skin. Menstruating women use an estimated twelve thousand tampons over their lifetime. It doesn't make any sense for a woman to insert into her vagina tampons that may contain traces of pesticide, month after month, year after year—and it's not just pesticide residues, which are linked to endocrine disruption and cancer, but also dioxins, allergens, fragrances, and parabens (preservatives). I use washable cloth pads, but please research alternatives to commercial tampon brands that will work for you.

## *Clothe the body*

OEKO-TEX is a certification standard for textiles and fabric items. Husband and I bought some sheets that were OEKO-TEX certified, and neither the sheets nor any part of the packaging had any toxic smell at all. I would expect standard sheets that were not certified in this way to have been very likely treated with pesticides and then also treated with a light fragrance to mask the smell of the pesticides. The warehouses storing the packages might be perfumed or the store is full of fragrance so that when you bring in the package, you are also bringing in the toxic fragrance. As much as you possibly can, avoid purchasing items that must be dry-cleaned.

I love the idea of thrift-shop clothing, but these items are inevitably impregnated with fragrance and sometimes impregnated with mothball residue. The tiniest leftover amount of mothballs makes me quite ill, even if I can't smell it, and, like thrift-shop fragrance, it is nearly impossible to get this chemical out of clothing, blankets, or other fabric items. I have noticed that often fleece clothing has a very slight but nasty chemical smell, and fleece items have made me ill in the past. I do not purchase any shoes that have a chemical smell coming from them.

Because I was made ill by a sleep mask that was constructed from light synthetic fabric fused to foam, I now don't trust standard bras that are made this way. The off-gassing from the toxic components in standard bras can enter your body through your lungs as you breathe near them. Also, your skin is absorptive. The chemicals are surely entering your body, right next to the lymph nodes in your breast and armpit area. I don't wear a bra from day to day and instead have sewn tops for myself that have either decorative stitching or appliqué across the bodice to obscure my nipples. If I go for a run, I wear a compression-type sports bra or layer two of them, but these bras seem safer to me because they don't have foam in them.

Overall, for linens, clothing, and shoes, I don't have an easy answer, except to suggest approaching each purchase with skepticism and caution. Use the items you currently own for as long as you can to avoid buying these toxic fabric items the way they are being treated now. When possible, buy organic from reputable sources.

## HOME

### *Clean the home*

The single most important step you can take to reduce the toxicity of your home is to use nonfragranced laundry products. Fragrances are insufficiently regulated, and their components are not required to be identified. Many of these components are known toxins, endocrine disruptors, and neuro-disruptors. For anyone with any degree of chemical sensitivity, fragranced laundry products are at the top of their list for triggers.

Manufacturers are touting how long their "fresh" scents last, and indeed these fragrances seem to have supernatural qualities of persistence. Try to train your mind to see these fragrances as bad for you, not as pleasant indicators of "freshness." There have been many studies that indicate that the air coming out of a dryer vent from laundry washed with standard products is highly toxic.

Regarding other cleaning products, I believe that much of the current mania for fragrance in cleaning products is due to the manufacturers' desire to mask the unpleasant aromas of underlying ingredients. It's also to train consumers that these smells mean "clean," when of course what they actually signify is toxic garbage. Whatever the underlying motivation for the prevalence of these fragrances, to protect yourself and your family I suggest *no* fragranced products.

### *Conduct home administration*

My go-to cartridge respirator is the 3M Half Facepiece Reusable Respirator. The cartridges are sold separately, and there are different cartridges for different airborne toxins. I use the 3M Multigas/Vapor Cartridge/Filter 60926. I also keep with me a simple carbon fabric filter mask, the 3M Particulate Respirator 8247, R95. I reach for a dust mask frequently, and my favorite is 3M Particulate Respirator 9211/37022 (AAD) N95. Husband and I use the Blueair Classic 203 room filter boxes with a carbon filter.

I keep a five-gallon bucket on the porch near the mailbox, and 95 percent of the mail volume goes directly into the bucket for recycling. I strip everything nonessential away from bills before I bring them inside. The pages that I do plan to bring inside are first spread out in a drafty three-season porch to air out. I wear my cartridge respirator when handling the mail initially and also when paying the bills. No catalogs, circulars, or magazines are *ever* brought into the house. I diligently get myself removed from catalog mailing lists by calling their 1-800 number and requesting this removal, and I have chosen paperless billing for many items. Both of these approaches work well to reduce the overall volume of toxic paper arriving in the mailbox in the first place.

I wear my cartridge mask when feeding the woodstoves because of gasses from the fire itself, which happen to affect me strongly. When we first had the woodstoves installed, we needed to run them at a high temperature for much longer than the manufacturer recommended to burn off the manufacturing residues and off-gas the epoxies. I also wear my cartridge mask when I am in the basement area that contains the gas burner for our heating system. I wear the mask when I'm unloading the dishwasher because of gasses that accumulate within the dishwasher. Even though the detergent is environmentally friendly, it still causes me trouble when superheated. I avoid the area of the dishwasher when it is running because of a smell that emanates that seems to be chlorine-based.

The elephant in the room is the current housing stock, built and/or renovated with toxic materials and, by now, also contaminated with fragranced products. If you plan to move because your own house is toxic in ways that cannot be corrected, be sure to research regional fracking. Fracking destroys water supplies.

### *Furnish the home*

I suggest that you empty out your bedroom as much as you can. Remove books, papers, plastic items, electronics, extra clothing and shoes, and extra fabric and foam items. In this way, you can create a safe haven inside your house as a transition toward a cleaner home overall.

Often lower-quality plastic items have a discernable smell, which is an indication that there are toxins present in the plastic. Try to find higher-quality nonstink items. Many plastic items are made in molds, and often it is the mold-release compounds that are making the worst smells. You can wash off these compounds and improve the safety of the items. Stay away from PVC. Polyethylene vinyl acetate (PEVA) is considered less toxic, and I have not had trouble with our PEVA shower curtain.

Most books are printed with inks that create toxic off-gassing. Even older books, meaning books that are twenty to thirty years old, can be toxic in my experience. Try to get as many books out of your living space as you can. Be careful with books around your small children. If there is a book I want to read, I take it outside on a breezy day and wear my respirator. I'm sure that books printed with nontoxic inks are an improvement, but I am not convinced yet just how nontoxic these inks are or what other toxins might still exist in the paper, glues, and other components. I did not have any trouble with my Kindle Paperwhite e-reader, but I was careful to leave all of its packaging outside and also to wipe down the surfaces of all of its cables and accessories with a light soap foam to remove the mold-release compounds.

Research nontoxic versions of electronic products before purchasing. EPEAT is a worldwide environmental and safety standard for electronic products, and Hewlett Packard has many products that satisfy either the EPEAT silver or the EPEAT gold standard. I found that company salespeople didn't know which models were in compliance with which standard, but when I insisted that they bear down and find out, they did. Hewlett Packard EPEAT gold computers have not made me sick.

Standard carpets and soft furnishings are made with an infinite and inadequately regulated cocktail of components such as dyes, preservatives, synthetic fibers, and glues. Look for nontoxic finishes and cushions without flame retardants such as boric acid and formaldehyde.

It is natural to want to fill your child's room with lovely products that express how much you care about your child, but this instinct is causing many people to inadvertently expose their young children to toxic materials. I recommend a spare approach, meaning few objects, given the overall toxicity of so many products. Each object should be carefully vetted. Also, the floor, wall, and ceiling surfaces must be extremely carefully considered, as well as light fixtures. This point is so vitally important that it cannot be overstated. If you must renovate or paint, use the least toxic materials you can find and be sure to air out the room for at least several weeks afterward.

## CAR

Approach your car as if it is dangerous, and be aware that you are entering a toxic zone. Do not subject your children to this space unnecessarily. Air the car out before you get in, and be especially attentive if the car has been in the sun on a hot day. The electrical and electronic components under the dashboard—like PVC coatings on wires, for example—will off-gas generally, but this will be much worse when they are heated by the sun. Drive for a minute with the windows open before turning on the air conditioning or the heating system so that gasses that have built up in these systems have a chance to escape to the outside. If the outside air quality is acceptable, try to keep fresh air coming in and adjust the vents to let in air. Before buying a car, research "nontoxic car interiors." Volvo has at least acknowledged the problem and identified the worst components. If your car manufacturer says there is not a problem, they are lying. If you think large car companies don't lie, remember the Volkswagen diesel-emissions scandal.

## OUT AND ABOUT

The whole purpose of this book is to encourage you to organize your life so that you stay home more. When you are considering going out, remember the port-a-potty and its evil cousins, airplane, train, and bus toilets. It is a certainty that these places, horrific with the stench of fragranced disinfectant and the sight of the bobbing turds and discarded menstrual products of strangers, are harming your children. If dropping your dirt in peace at home is the apotheosis of enlightenment and dignity, then port-a-potties are the epitome of degradation and denial. Humankind should develop a reasonable alternative to the port-a-potty rather than give money to children who think that they could or should travel to Mars. When I have to use a port-a-potty, I feel like I am entering hell. First, I take several deep breaths outside and upwind to oxygenate my blood, and then I don my mask and try to breathe as little as possible while inside the stinky, disgusting toilet-box. Ironically, being panicked and oxygen-deprived makes my internal organs relax deeply, as if I'm about to shit on myself—not a happy picture and another reason to just stay home.

# About the Author

Pookie Sekmet grew up in the US South and went to Harvard College before becoming a computer professional and later an accountant. She has been happily married for about thirty years, and lives in a small town in Western Massachusetts. As a baby, she suffered a chemical exposure that her parents hid from her and that triggered a lifelong and undiagnosed intolerance to common chemicals. *Sensitive* is the story of how she solved the central mystery of why she had been ill from an early age, worked out ways of avoiding chemical reinjury, and accepted the true nature of her birth family.

# Selected Titles from She Writes Press

She Writes Press is an independent publishing company founded to serve women writers everywhere. Visit us at www.shewritespress.com.

*Not a Poster Child: Living Well with a Disability—A Memoir* by Francine Falk-Allen. $16.95, 978-1631523915. Francine Falk-Allen was only three years old when she contracted polio and temporarily lost the ability to stand and walk. Here, she tells the story of how a toddler learned grown-up lessons too soon; a schoolgirl tried her best to be a "normie," on into young adulthood; and a woman finally found her balance, physically and spiritually.

*Raw* by Bella Mahaya Carter. $16.95, 978-1-63152-345-8. In an effort to holistically cure her chronic stomach problems, Bella Mahaya Carter adopted a 100 percent raw, vegan diet—a first step on a quest that ultimately dragged her, kicking and screaming, into spiritual adulthood.

*Body 2.0: Finding My Edge Through Loss and Mastectomy* by Krista Hammerbacher Haapala. An authentic, inspiring guide to reframing adversity that provides a new perspective on preventative mastectomy, told through the lens of the author's personal experience.

*Beautiful Affliction: A Memoir* by Lene Fogelberg. $16.95, 978-1-63152-985-6. The true story of a young woman's struggle to raise a family while her body slowly deteriorates as the result of an undetected fatal heart disease.

*Not by Accident: Reconstructing a Careless Life* by Samantha Dunn. $16.95, 978-1-63152-832-3. After suffering a nearly fatal riding accident, lifelong klutz Samantha Dunn felt compelled to examine just what it was inside herself—and other people—that invited carelessness and injury.

*The Great Healthy Yard Project: Our Yards, Our Children, Our Responsibility* by Diane Lewis, MD. $24.95, 978-1-938314-86-5. A comprehensive look at the ways in which we are polluting our drinking water and how it's putting our children's future at risk—and what we can do to turn things around.

www.ingramcontent.com/pod-product-compliance
Lightning Source LLC
Chambersburg PA
CBHW021621301224
19582CB00009B/71

9 781631 526183